What is the HCG + 500 Weight Loss Cure?

The **HCG + 500 Calorie** 'protocol,' as it's discoverer, **Dr. A.T.W. Simeons** called it, is an amazing, but as yet unheralded, discovery for the **treatment** and **veritable cure** of **'obesity.'** HCG is the mercifully short acronym for the tongue twisting, scientific name for the hormone **Human Chorionic Gonadotrophin.**

The **HCG discovery began** when the good doctor made this shrewd observation...

"...refusing to be side tracked by the all too facile interpretation of obesity, I have always held that overeating is the RESULT of the disorder, not it's CAUSE..."

The **HCG hormone** in your system, **safely causes the loss of weight** by activating your warehoused **'abnormal fat'** back into circulation where it can be accessed.

Adding to the protocol, a **Caloric intake of only 500 Calories daily,** under a **strict but simple plan of eating**, results in your body consuming your **'abnormal warehoused fat,'** to **make up the balance** of it's **daily Caloric needs.**

"This normally results in weight loss of about a pound a day on average."

If you **follow the plan** carefully, **as prescribed** by Dr. Simeons, **you can achieve:**

- **Excellent Appetite Control**
- **Weight Loss Averaging About a Pound a Day**
- **Elimination of Inches of 'Warehoused Fat'**
- **Beneficial Health Results as a Side Effect!**
- **Steady and Rapid Decline of Your Obesity.**

"Thus it is possible to leave your 'good' fat untouched and burn up your 'bad' fat."

You Can Defeat & Control Obesity Forever with the 'HCG + 500 Calorie Protocol'

Endorsements from HCG Weight Loss Cure 'Alumni'

"...it is easy to see from the **results** I am getting that **Dr. Simeons** really **knew his stuff...**"

"...I kept an open mind, did everything as perfect as I could, and experienced **eye-popping results**, in less than **63 days**... **I lost 55 pounds**."

"**You will see** if you follow the protocol... that **this is the real deal**."

"When **understood correctly**, this HCG program is **not** a **weight loss program**, rather it is a once and for all **'cure for obesity...'**"

Absolutely **nothing I've ever tried** has been this **effective** or this **easy**. I **lost 35 pounds** so easily I felt like I was somehow cheating..."

"In my opinion, the **HCG assisted diet protocol** is a genuine **medical marvel**!"

"...HCG is **not a drug**; rather it is a **natural human hormone** that our body 'knows' exactly how to use..."

"...I **lost 100 pounds** in about **90 days** and am keeping it off...

"I **saw the results** with the **HCG diet** and decided to try it. I continued my exercise program... and **shocked my trainer** when the results came back."

"Great program, **easy**, and **it works**."

You Have Found the Genuine Answer... ...HCG and the 'HCG Diet Victory Collection.'

Acknowledgements & Thanks.

Special Acknowledgement.

I would like to acknowledge and thank my very own personal physician for sharing the work of Dr. Simeons with me in my quest for a better quality of life, free of obesity and it's debilitating complications. If you looked up the definition of 'enlightened physician,' her picture would be there.

Thank You.

Many thanks to you dear reader, for making the 'HCG Victory Collection' a best seller among the HCG diet books. Thank you also for investing your money and trust and faith in the content, I appreciate it. I work very hard to make it valuable.

I have worked long and hard and poured my heart & soul into this book. This planner will always have a special place in my heart as I worked on it during my mother's final days on this earth.

As some famous author once said,
"...it was the best of times and it was the worst of times..."

I have done my best for you. It was a great adventure and now I plan to go have another one, as I work to complete my 'HCG Diet Victory Recipe' book, brought to you as they say, 'in living color.' Finally, I thank my wife for her patience.

Your Feedback is Appreciated.

If you have questions, concerns or input for me, contact me at the email below. I may not be able to personally answer every email, due to time constraints, as my wife and I are care givers in our home, for my youngest daughter Jessica, who was totally disabled at age 3 months by her vaccinations. However, I do read and value all feedback, whether it is positive or negative, and will address it in the appropriate venue to the best of my ability.

email: HCGDietBoise@gmail.com

It is the desire of my heart that you experience complete victory.

JIM :]

You Have Found the Genuine Answer... ...HCG and the 'HCG Diet Victory Collection.'

Comments and Reviews
about the 'HCG Diet Victory Collection.'

" I LOVE the **pre-made EZPlans™**...this planner
saves a tremendous amount of **time**
and **eliminates** the **confusion** out there..."

"I keep track of everything using my **trusty charts** in
my **HCG Victory book**! Yea! I love them!"

" ...if **Doctor Simeons** were alive today he **would love** this fresh
and **simple presentation** of his concepts..."

"Foods **that may be** consumed... are outlined, and foods
that **may not be eaten** are **not mentioned**.
That **decreases confusion** among my **clients**."

"...another **remarkably simple** and **straight forward**
guide to **success** with this HCG diet program."

"...**Dr. Simeons would be proud**...
keep up the **great work**!"

...**you shouldn't fail** if you follow the **plan** and
use the tools... a really fine job."

"...I love the **up-beat & positive** aspects..."

"**...this is exactly what I needed**... a
streamlined set of tools for **maximizing**
my success & minimizing the confusion..."

You Have Found the Genuine Answer...
...HCG and the 'HCG Victory Collection.'

HCG DIET VICTORY MASTER PLANNER

*If some way...can be found
to cope effectively with this
universal problem
of modern civilized man,
our world will be a happier
place for countless
fellow men and women."*

Dr. A. T. W. Simeons

Defeat OBESITY...Forever!

The HCG Assisted 500 Calorie Weight Loss Cure

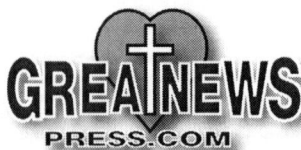

GREATNEWS PRESS.COM

www.greatnewspress.com

Inspirational Books
Diet. Health & Nutrition

Introduction: **CONTENTS Quick OVERVIEW**

©HCGDietVictoryPlanner.com 8 ISBN 978-0-9800641-8-6

Introduction: CONTENTS Detail

Dedication: A.T.W. Simeons

A Brief Summary of the Life of 'The Einsein of Obesity.'..11

Introduction: 'Congratulation & Welcome'

You Have Chosen Wisely, The 'HCG Victory Collection,' What Would Dr. Simeons Say? 13
Lowering the Bar.,Keeping it Simple.As Simple as 1... 2... 3.
Worry Free HCG Diet EZPlans™, 'Poof' It Works Like Magic..15
Something Worth Repeating... Lose it Sooner... Not Later!..16

SECTION ONE: 'Taking the First Step'

Making the Most of this Planner, The First Step, Meeting the Challenges,
Reader Feedback: Topics of Interest & Concern 19
Answering the Questions as Simply As Possible,
Step 1. Physician's Exam & Testing 20
Step 2. Education & Study,
Step 3. 500 Calories + HCG,
Step 4. Weight Setting the 'No Sugar - No Starch' Way. 21
Step 5. Returning to Normal,
Step 5a. Unique New Options: Discovering Your
Metabolism Blueprint™
Step 6. Maintaining Your Specific Daily Food Needs..22

HCG + 500 Calories: BRIEF REVIEW

Reviewing the 500 Calorie + HCG Weight Loss Plan, Entering The World of 'Fat Facts.'
HCG Defined..25
The Bottom Line.,Don't Be Afraid... But Do Choose Wisely, Dr. Simeons 500 Calorie Plan. 26
Breakfast: Lunch: Dinner: Condiments & Seasonings: Drinks & Fluid Intake:................................27
A Convenient Refresher Course, A Closer Look at the Diet Plan.
Do Not Exceed 500 Calories per Day, Dr. Simeons did the 'Heavy Lifting.'
Remember: Rotating Your Protein Selection of is Critical..28

HCG 'Immunitiy' & 'Shots'

Water Water Everywhere. ALL NEW Six Day 'Pre-Made EZPlans™' Save Time & Confusion,
'HOT BUTTON' the 'HCG Immunity Syndrome,' HCG in the 21st Century. 29
The Bottom Line: An Even Faster Result, Okay, Let's Talk About Needles.Ouch!
Here's Why I Don't Like the 'Shots' Scene, Here are my Reasons:..30

HCG "Starting Out Right"

Don't Forget to 'Gorge Yourself,' Existing Health Concerns and
Common Sense, Beneficial Side Effects Can Result. 31

HCG + 500 Calories: 'Groceries'

Loading the Chuck Wagon, CAUTION: Always Check the INGREDIENTS. 35
Grocery Shopping Time, Food Group 1: Proteins for Victory, Food Group 2: Vegetables for Victory,
Food Group 3: Fruits for Victory, Food Group 4: 'Starches' for Victory 36
Walk on the Wild Side, Wild Card Group: Beverages:
SWEETENERS... If You Can't Live Without Them. 37

HCG + 500 Calorie EZPlans™

Introducing 'HCG EZPlans™' Handy Pre-Made 6 Day Food Plans.
What are 'HCG EZPlans?'..39
Nutritional Information on 500 Calorie Choices & Options. 40
Pre-made 500 Calorie EZPlans™..41-43
Blank EZPLan™ 500 Calorie Forms..45-51

Introduction: CONTENTS Detail

Introduction: CONTENTS Detail

Reference for Tables: 'HCG Diet Victory PLANNER'

Dedication:

Dr. A.T.W. Simeons

"The 'Einstein' of obesity."

Please read a brief summary about the 'Einstein of obesity.'

Born in London, Dr. Simeons graduated summa cum laude from the University of Heidelberg with a medical degree. He completed his post-graduate studies in Germany and Switzerland was appointed to a hospital near Dresden.

Eventually he became engrossed in the study of tropical diseases, 'malaria' in particular, which led him to join the 'School of Tropical Medicine' in Hamburg.

Following two years of work in Africa, he went to India in 1931. He found himself so fascinated by the country and its health problems that he stayed for eighteen years. He discovered the use of injectable 'atebrin' for malaria and was awarded a Red Cross Order of Merit, for his new 'Simeons Stain,' method of 'staining' malaria parasites to identify them, which is still being used today

During World War II, he held several important Government posts in India, conducting extensive research on bubonic plague and leprosy control, and founding a model 'leper colony' which today is an all-India center.

"... founding a model 'leper colony' which is now an all-India center."

He set up in private practice in Bombay for a time and then, with his wife and three sons, moved to Rome in 1949. Working on his new interest, 'psychosomatic disorders,' at the Salvator Mundi International Hospital.

Dr. Simeons also authored several medical books as well as, contributing to many scientific publications and journals. His life ended in 1970.

The 'HCG Diet Victory Collection' is gratefully dedicated to all of his brilliant work.

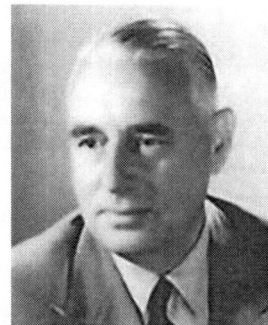

I can tell from studying his writings, that I would have liked Dr. Simeons a lot. It's a shame we never met. He strikes me as a dedicated, humble and unpretentious man, who had a genuine concern for the less fortunate. Through his medical research and study, he spent his life helping people. No baloney... just results.

I for one, am grateful. He was a 'cut to the chase' kind of guy with common sense. We need more like him. In his matter of fact way he understood, and accepted the irony of solving a less glamourous problem, when he wistfully wrote the following...

"The 'HCG Victory Collection' is gratefully dedicated to his brilliant work."

"The problems of obesity are perhaps not so dramatic as the problems of cancer, or polio, but they often cause life long suffering."

He knew he would be ignored, and yet he did all the unglamorous, painstaking work anyway. He was doing it for you and for me, and the untold numbers of people whose lives have been altered for the better, because of his brilliant work.

Thank You, Dr. Simeons.

Introduction: **'Congratulations & Welcome!'**

You Have Chosen Wisely.

For over 40 years, Dr. Simeons **dedicated his life,** to grappling with a very unglamorous subject... obesity. What he discovered is, in my opinion, a complete medical marvel. I am **still amazed,** as are many others, who are 'fat free' at last.

I was almost 65 years of age, the last 20 spent **struggling with obesity** and trying to it defeat it... with everything I had! Instead of winning the battle, my health and life expectancy slowly dwindled away.

I finally found **the answer.** You are at the gateway, that I passed through to victory.

The answer I found is 'Human Chorionic Gonadotrophin' which we shall simply call **HCG** from this point forward. Difficult to pronounce and not exactly accurately named. It really doesn't matter if you can say it... **HCG is amazing** and it works.

The 'HCG Victory Collection.'

As I experienced my **HCG diet,** I was fortunate to work with an **enlightened physician** who had been **properly trained** in the HCG assisted diet protocol.

I was struck by **an interesting contrast.** On the one hand was Doctor Simeons **pure and simple manuscript** and my personal doctors **clear direction,** on the other hand were the existing books on the subject, which were much more **complex & confusing** than necessary.

To compensate, **I waded through the confusion** and developed my own methods, forms and menus. One day my doctor saw my work, and said, **"You should write a book..."** From that seed, **a series of 'victory' books** has grown.

My background is in marketing-communications, graphics design and writing so it was the natural thing to do. From the very outset, I imagined **Dr. Simeons** as **my client** and although I have consulted with other **top experts** in the world, I still consider him **my inspiration** and try to **conform to his original prescription.**

What Would Dr. Simeons Say?

That's the question I constantly ask myself. Making **his light shine brighter** is my goal. He has done all of the hard stuff. With the patience of Job, he has sorted everything out. Really the whole thing is **very simple** and **almost foolproof** if you follow his plan **precisely** as he prescribed it.

Some **criticize his work** because of the lack of 'clinical studies.' I guess that means no rats were involved. To me that is **one of the strengths** of his method. He worked with painstaking trial and error with **human beings.**

He took the time to get to know them and to counsel them and listen to their stories. By his own admission a process that took **at least 40 years.**

Personally, I will take that kind of **large, long and in-depth experience** with people that could **articulate the experience,** before I would choose the results of a short term 'clinical study' with a bunch of lab rats.

On the **next page** is a simple **diagram** of Dr. Simeons' **'HCG diet Protocol.'**

"You have chosen to break free..."

"You are on the road to increasing vitality and health."

"HCG is amazing and it works."

Introduction: **The 'HCG Protocol' FLOW CHART**

"You will journey where you have never been before and discover many new things."

Mission Control

Enlightened Doctor
Medical History
'HCG Victory Tool Kit'
'HCG Diet PLANNER'
Goal & Target setting
HCG RX & Lab Tests
Follow Ups
Course Corrections
Consultations

500 Calorie Menu

HCG RX

20 day HCG course begins — 'Blast-off'

'Gorge' 2 Days — 'Extra Fuel on board' 2 DAYS

Course Correction 'Apple Day*'

Repeat HCG + 500 C. — 'Orbiting' 20 to 183 DAYS

Course Correction 'Steak Day*'

'Weight Setting' NO SUGAR/STARCH — 'Re-entry' 21 DAYS

Return to Normal Slowly add sugar & starches if desired — 'Return to Earth' 21 DAYS

"It is not without a cost, but if you stay the course you will return to earth a changed person and you will leave the fat behind... forever."

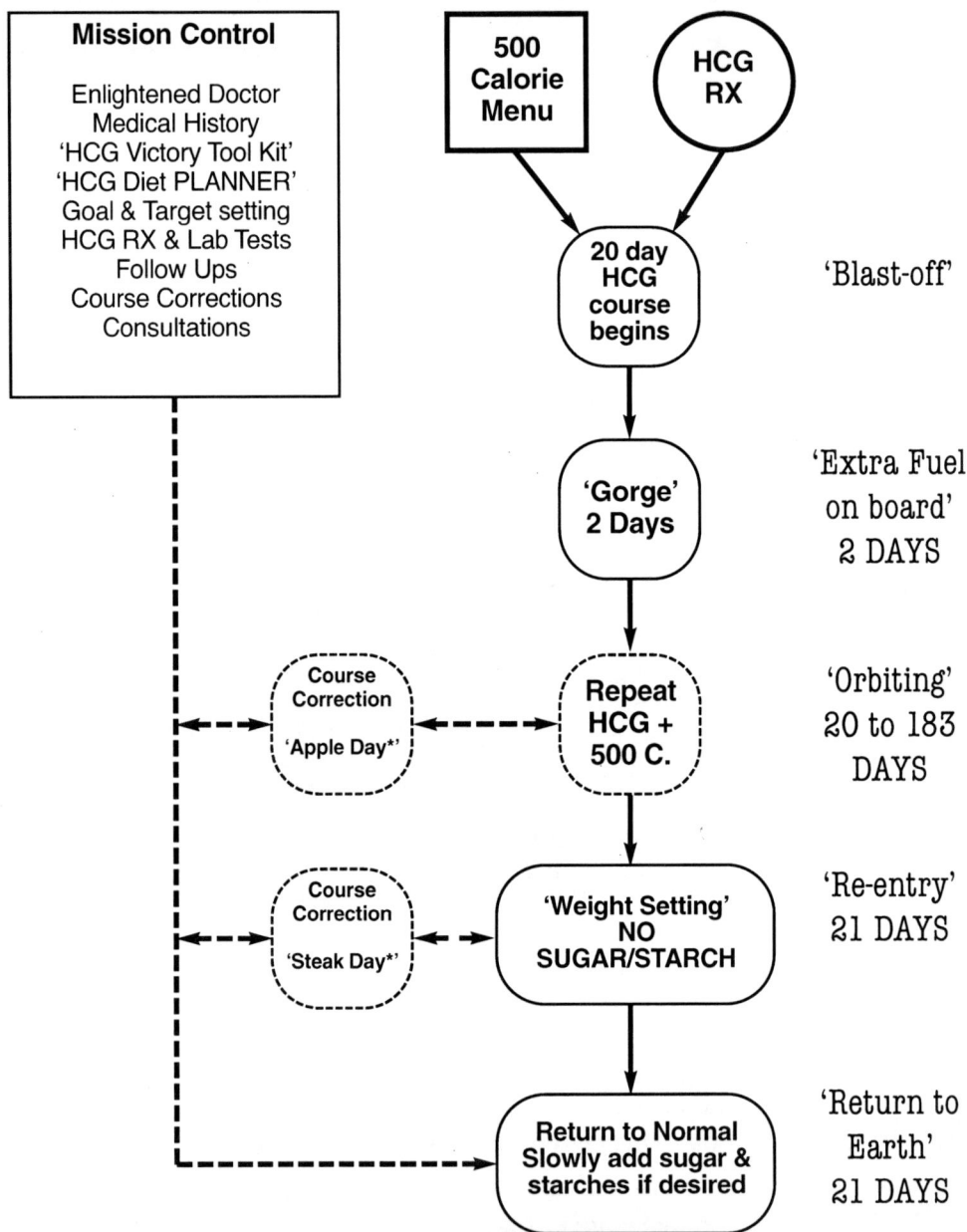

Table 1: The HCG Tool Kit Flow Chart of the Entire Protocol.

'The NO Sugar No Starch Zone' is the 'Weight Setting' step.

The **'Weight Setting'** step in the process is a major emphasis of this planner, along with some unique guidance and fresh ideas, to help you succeed long term. Use of this planner will save you time and facilitate your **permanent weight loss** solution.

More exact details on the use of the **'apple day'** and **'steak day** are covered as well as other tips are found in **Appendix C: 'Troubleshooting.'**

Introduction: **As Simple as Possible.**

"Why throw away all of the good old doctor's painstaking trial and error and his lifetime of refining, and add a bunch of unnecessary steps, and complications?"

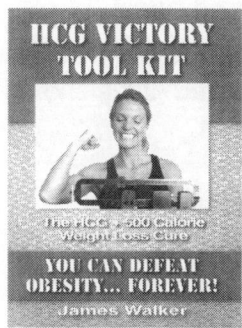

Lowering the Bar.

The HCG Diet really is simple. It is **simple** and straightforward **but very precise**.

Why throw away all of the good old doctor's **painstaking trial and error** and lifetime of **refining** and add a bunch of unnecessary steps and complications?

Why should we **obsess** about the unimportant?

Why not keep it **simple and focus** on the **critical essence** of the method?

Why not make it as **easy and accessible** as humanly possible?

What would Dr. Simeons do? I think I know.

That is **the inspiration** for all **of my books** on the subject. Let's make it **simple**.

Keeping it Simple.

The objective of this '**HCG Diet Victory Planner,**' and my purpose in creating it, is to **simplify** the whole thing. As I have stated before, I am not a fitness guru, or a nutrition expert or a doctor. But **I know the truth** when I see it. This is the **real deal**.

I am **not much different than you**, tired of the obesity battle and **frustrated** with all of the **extra fat** I was 'warehousing.'

I want to **share** theis solution with as many people as I can as fast as I can.

Like Dr. Simeons says "...the problems of obesity are not so dramatic as the problems of cancer or polio, but they often cause life long suffering." If you knew a cure for cancer that really worked and worked for everyone, could you keep it a secret?

As Simple as 1... 2... 3.

My first book the '**HCG Victory Tool Kit**' is **streamlined and simplified**. It is easier not harder. It is **focused on the essence** of the method that we all need to master to **optimize** our success. As old Albert Einstein often said, "... the solution should be no more difficult than it needs to be..." and "... the **solution** when found will be **simple**."

Worry Free HCG Diet EZPlans™

The **first step** is to **understand and carry out** the **HCG + 500 Calorie** part of the plan. Dr. Simeons said understanding the process is **a key to success**.

The '**HCG Victory Tool Kit**' contains a careful explanation of the **concepts** and the **tools**, **tips** and **record** keeping **forms** you need to be **victorious**. And as a **bonus** also contains a copy of **Dr. Simeon's original manuscript**, presented in **a fresh easy** to reference and read **form**. A complete introductory guide **for HCG dieting success**.

This follow-up book is a response to the **many people who requested** some time saving ways to **develop** and **quickly** put to use **a worry free menu plan** for both the **HCG + 500 step** and the **No Sugar/No Starch Weight Setting step**.

The most frequent feedback was "I am too busy to work up all of these eating plans..." They asked for a '**turn-key**' solution. They wanted **pre-made daily menu guides** that were **already figured out and ready to use**.

"... too busy to work up all of these eating plans..."

Introduction: Let's Keep it as Simple as Possible.

That is one of the the purposes of this planner. I call them **HCG Diet EZPLANS.**™

They are a series of **prepared eating guides suggested** for use in both the **500 Calorie + HCG step** and the **No Sugar/No Starch step.**

To start you will find **6 day plans** designed for the **500 calorie daily target.**

Then for the **No Sugar or Starch** step there are **6 day plans** in **100 Calorie** increments from **1200 all the way to 2600 Calorie targets. A real time saver.**

Plus you will find a supply of **blank menu** planning forms, as well as forms for **record keeping**, helps and tips and an **expanded appendix** for **review** and **reference.** Emphasis is on providing clear concise examples for maximum time savings.

'Poof' It Works Like Magic.

One of the most **amazing** things about this HCG plan is that it **works so quickly.**

As I have shared before, I lowered my weight by **22 pounds**, and my **blood sugar** by **139 points**, without medication... in the **first week.** Others have reported similar results, some even better. Dr. Simeons claim of 'on average loss of about a pound a day,' does repeatedly hold true.

Most women typically don't lose as fast or as much daily as men, but reach their goals, just the same. **Women** have other **biological influences** at work, as well as, the use of oils and cosmetics. Not to mention massages, manicures and pedicures!

You will experience **plateaus** and temporary set backs, but the pay off is there if you persevere. You will be **amazed** at your final result. We **all are amazed** at the end!

Something Worth Repeating... Lose it Sooner... Not Later!

Rapid feedback is one of the perks and helps **to keep you motivated.**

When I reviewed my first week results, I knew that **I had found the answer** I had been looking for. Here was something that worked exactly like it was supposed to.

It was **easy to stay motivated** and to pay the 'price' because I could sense that the reward was worth it. I was right.

I lost **55** pounds in **63 days** and I found a permanent solution. I had the magic bullet. Obesity in my life is now in the past. I am free from the chains of obesity and the multiple prescriptions. My blood sugar is now normal.

Today I **easily maintain** my weight, I eat better than I ever have, and I eat loads of nutritious, delicious and healthy foods, I don't walk around hollow eyed and hungry.

I am FREE.

You will be too. Just **go for it!**

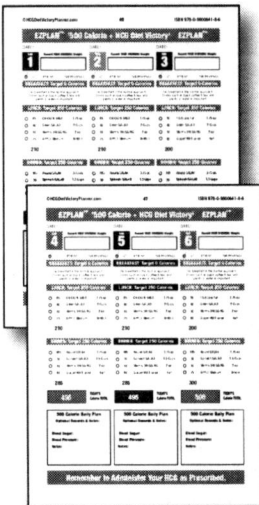

"One of the most amazing things about this HCG plan is that it works so quickly."

"It was easy to stay motivated..."

Section One:

'Taking the First Step.'

*"The journey of
a thousand miles
begins with
a single step."*

Chinese Proverb

Defeat OBESITY...Forever!

The HCG Assisted 500 Calorie Weight Loss Cure

Section One: **'Taking the First Step'**

Making the Most of this Planner.

One of my doctor's favorite sayings is, " I am the **options** person... I will explain all of them to you... I will help you, but **you must decide**, which option is right for you."

Isn't that a **refreshing attitude**? And after all, isn't that the way it should be?

A sense of **cooperation** and **understanding** between a **doctor and a patient**, what **a shocking concept** in this age of 'modern' medicine. After years of dealing with haughty, dictatorial doctors who seem to ooze a sense of entitlement, hearing my doctor say that for the first time, was a **breath of fresh air**.

That's one of the **guiding inspirations** for this **planner**. To give you **options** and **guides** to show you how to **maximize** your experience and to help **you decide** the **correct course** for you... as **simply, clearly** and **efficiently** as possible.

The First Step.

If a journey of a thousand miles **begins with one step**. That one step should be in the **right direction**. Assembled in this planner you will find a number of important steps for achieving **maximum victory** with Dr. Simeons HCG weight loss method.

Some of the steps must be very **measured** and very tightly **controlled,** and then a little less so, and finally a gradual release, to complete freedom. So in this planner you will find those scenarios laid out for you. At **each step** along the way you will see **freedom gradually increasing** but always **under your control.**

You will see **guides** that give you a **clear concise picture** of the available options.

Meeting the Challenges.

Preparing a book like this one is full of challenges. The realization that **I might never please everyone** was **outweighed** by the **hope and desire** that I could **help as many as possible** by making **a unique contribution.**

Many **successful HCG dieters** are using the first volume in this series, the '**HCG Victory Tool Kit,**' to successfully **complete the diet**. Some are looking to maximize their new found **success** now and in the future, and **moving on** to a 'normal' **eating lifestyle**, incorporating newly acquired, healthier food selections.

Others are just starting the **HCG diet** and are looking for **a clear path to success.**

Reader Feedback: Topics of Interest & Concern.

Looking back at the **feedback** and the **most common questions** received, a definite pattern emerges. Here are the **top three topics** requested:

1. "Can you give me a list of **pre-made food choices** and **eating options**?"

2. "How can I easily incorporate the **non-dieting members** of my family?"

3. "Dr. Simeons says very little about, **returning to normal**... any suggestions?"

There are **other concerns** that are more specific, such as 'shots' & 'immunity.' These issues will be **addressed and examined** in more depth in this book.

"...you must decide, which option is right for you."

"That one step, should be in the right direction."

"... I might never please everyone... ...outweighed by the hope and desire that I could help as many as possible..."

Section One: **'Taking the First Step'**

"Keeping the focus on being clear & simple..."

Answering the Questions as Simply As Possible.

Keeping the focus on **being clear and simple** with a minimum amount of mumbo jumbo I have spent a huge amount of time **researching and examining** the areas of feedback just listed.

Below is an overall diagram of the **progression** through the steps of the **HCG diet protocol**. I know it has become popular to refer to the 'phases' as popularized by other authors, but I choose to take **a fresh approach** that is more in-line with Doctor Simeons **original prescription**. (see **Table 2** below)

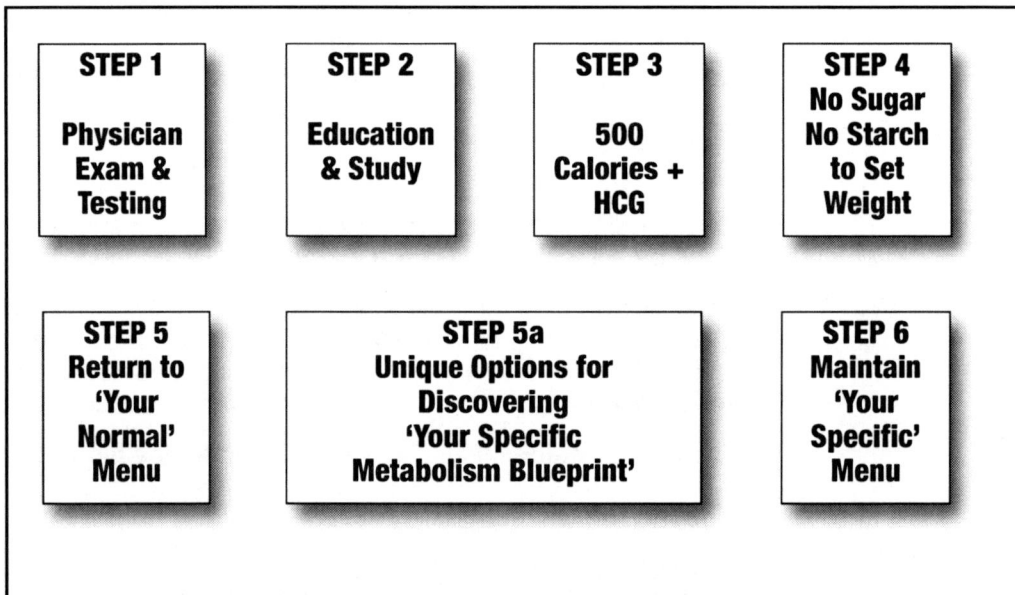

STEP 1 Physician Exam & Testing	STEP 2 Education & Study	STEP 3 500 Calories + HCG	STEP 4 No Sugar No Starch to Set Weight
STEP 5 Return to 'Your Normal' Menu	STEP 5a Unique Options for Discovering 'Your Specific Metabolism Blueprint'		STEP 6 Maintain 'Your Specific' Menu

Table 2: 'Overview of the Ideal HCG Success Plan'

STEP 1

Physician Exam & Testing

Step 1. Physician's Exam & Testing

To do the **HCG assisted weight loss protocol** the way it's **author and creator designed it**, you should take this **important first step**. Yes, I know on the internet, there all kinds of self appointed 'hcg diet experts' advising people to skip this step, and even advising how to do it. Not a good approach in my opinion.

In fact, I find this **compromising attitude,** sad and **amazingly irresponsible**.

I **am not** one of those people and **never** will be. The advice I am going to give you will **always be consistent & conforming** to the **original prescription**. And also conforming, to the instruction of the **world's most qualified** HCG doctors & clinics.

As Doctor Simeons emphasized, *" Any patient who thinks he can reduce by taking a few 'shots' and eating less is not only sure to be disappointed but may be heading for serious trouble."* I don't think it could be any plainer.

Let's **stay true** to his **instructions**, **stay out of trouble** and **maximize** the benefits.

STEP 2 **Education & Study**

Step 2. Education & Study

One of the **keys to maximizing your success** and good health is to **understand** and **participate** in the process. One of the **reasons for this planner** and the **'HCG Victory Tool Kit,'** is to facilitate that as **painlessly as possible.**

To that end, and as a matter of **convenience**, you will find a few **reviews** included throughout this book. Sometimes it helps to have **a brief review** to stay on course, especially if it has been a while **since your initial HCG course** of treatment.

But in any case, **you will do better** all the way around if you keep your brain engaged. Remember according to Dr. Simeons, **the secret to obesity control** really is **in your head.** Certainly true in more ways than one.

STEP 3 **500 Calories + HCG**

Step 3. 500 Calories + HCG

This is the **original Dr. Simeons HCG protocol.** You will find a **review** and **brief explanations**, exact **food groups**, as well as **menu guides** and **forms.**

A new **time saving feature** of this planner, is **pre-made 6 day eating guides.**

Tucked away in the **appendix** are a few **additional tools** and **helpful information.**

STEP 4 **No Sugar** **No Starch** **to Set** **Weight**

Step 4. Weight Setting the 'No Sugar - No Starch' Way.

Once you have **achieved your weight goals** you begin the process of **setting that weight,** as your new 'normal,' in your **brain's control system.** (see **Section Two**)

Once again the old doctor did all of the hard stuff. The **correct procedure** is worked out for you. What **you need to do** is to determine your **Caloric needs** and to **follow an eating plan** that prohibits **sugars and starches** and allows a broader but **very precise food group** selection.

To keep that process as **clear and easy** as possible, in this planner you will find a number of **handy and time saving guides,** featuring **plenty of options.**

First you will find on **pages 57-61,** a simple method of determing **your Caloric needs.** This facilitates setting up **your daily Calorie targets.**

"...a large selection of pre-made plans to guide you..."

Once you have your Calorie targets you need **a daily plan** to achieve and monitor them. To address that issue I have included a large section of **pre-made plans** to guide you. They start at **1200** and run to **2600 Calories** in **100 Calorie** increments. Once again these are designed **to guide you** and **save time.** You also will find plenty of **blank forms** for writing your own **personalized plans.**

The pre-made **EZPlans™ cover 6 days.** This allows for the insertion of a **'steak day'** or just a **repeat** of **your favorite day,** to fill out the week. They are also designed to be **mixed** and **matched** using **odd and even** days. This will allow you to continue the **practice prescribed** by Dr. Simeons of **alternating your protein choices.** Something that by now, should seem normal to you, and in your routine. Lots of **flexibility,** but **under control,** and **streamlined** to save time.

Simply **repeat the plan** until you have **set your weight** and completed this step, and you are **ready to move on** to the next step... **'Returning to Normal.'**

**STEP 5
Return to
'Your
Normal'
Menu**

Step 5. Returning to Normal

Dr. Simeons had very little to say on this subject. It does seem logical, that perhaps he had **ideas left unexpressed,** that he never published.

One of the **issues to address** is just exactly **what is 'normal.'** Curious about precisely that question, I did some **research**. My own observations have been, that there does seem to be a **different 'normal' for different people.**

The **fruits of my research** resulted in some **very interesting discoveries**, that confirmed the fact, that **individual metabolism types** do exist and their **basic needs can be somewhat different**.

The concepts uncovered are based on over **80 years of research**, by a number of brilliant **physicians and scientists**. I think their work confirms and also describes, a fairly simple way to find, what I shall call, your **'metabolic blueprint.'**

Interestingly the pioneers of this discovery were **contemporaries** of Dr. Simeons, since the **original research** began in the 1930's.

It is noteworthy that many of the food choices identified are **very selective** and **reminiscent** of Dr. Simeons carefully constructed **food groups**. That makes me wonder if he was **aware of this concept,** which was emerging, when he was doing his **original obesity research**. Impossible to know for sure, but plausible.

**STEP 5a

A Unique
'Metabolism
Blueprint'**

Step 5a. Unique New Options: Discovering Your Metabolism Blueprint™

One of the **curiosities** that strikes you when you are first exposed to Dr. Simeons meticulously chosen food groups, is why his experience and trial and error over forty years, indicated that **some foods work well and some don't.**

The concept of **individual metabolism** may give us a clue. This concept is an extension of the physical **individuality** that is not only self evident, but readily and universally acknowledged. We are all the same in many ways, and yet definitely **individually unique.** I can visualize it as a blueprint. Not just any blueprint but a 'one-off' **custom blueprint.** Just like 'Tigger.' **you are the only one of your kind.**

You don't have to look very far to see that. Your **fingerprints** for instance. Experts can, by carefully examining your unique set of fingerprints, determine **exactly** who you are **out of billions** of individuals on this planet. Another example would be **DNA research,** which has scientically confirmed that **every hair** on your head is **uniquely yours**. Quite literally, the hairs on your head, are numbered.

Much **more on this concept** and it's impact on your new normal in **Section Three.**

**STEP 6
Maintain
'Your
Specific'
Menu**

Step 6. Maintaining Your Specific Daily Food Needs

Once you have your **'metabolism blueprint'** and have set-up your new personal normal you need to **monitor** and **periodically adjust it** as your lifestyle factors, such as age, occupation, location and goals change. You **don't need to obsess on this,** but your **unique normal** is **impacted** to some degree **by external factors**.

We'll look at this **ongoing maintenance & more resources** in **Section Three.**

HCG + 500 CALORIES

BRIEF REVIEW

BRIEF REVIEW · HCG + 500

Section One:

HCG + 500 Calories: BRIEF REVIEW

STEP 2

Education & Study

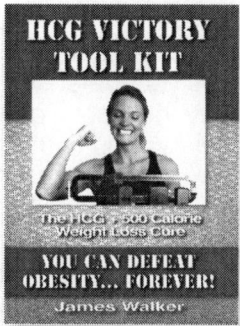

HCG VICTORY TOOL KIT

The HCG + 500 Calorie Weight Loss Cure

YOU CAN DEFEAT OBESITY... FOREVER!

James Walker

The HCG Victory Tool Kit ©2009

"What is indisputable is that Dr. Simeons research and testing has unlocked an incredible technique..."

"Activation by the HCG of the abnormal fat puts it back into circulation where it is consumed..."

Reviewing the 500 Calorie + HCG Weight Loss Plan

A quick review is **helpful,** both for those of you who are new to the weight loss method, and the HCG alumni who are returning for a tune-up. For those of you wanting an **in-depth explanation** or to read **Dr. Simeons original instructions,** Please refer to the 'HCG Victory Tool Kit.' This is important for your success.

What is indisputable, is that Dr. Simeons research and **testing has unlocked an incredible technique,** harnessing **natural body processes,** to **eliminate** and **control** abnormal or **'warehoused fat.'** His technique utilizes at least two natural weight management functions. First is the **fat mobilizing effects** of HCG and the second is the **effect of a very low calorie food intake.**

Entering The World of 'Fat Facts.'

First and foremost, we have **three kinds of fat**:

1) **'structural fat'** (good and necessary)
2) **'dynamic fat'** (our reserve fat fuel 'checking account')
3) **'static fat'** (bad fat and **the source of our obesity,** our 'fat warehouse')

The **'static fat'** is **dead weight** and will normally remain in our body's warehouse. We must do something about it **specifically** or we cannot win the battle.

Master Weight Control System.

Our brain's **weight control center** monitors and controls the movement of fat in our body and is responsible for the **excess fat warehousing** function.

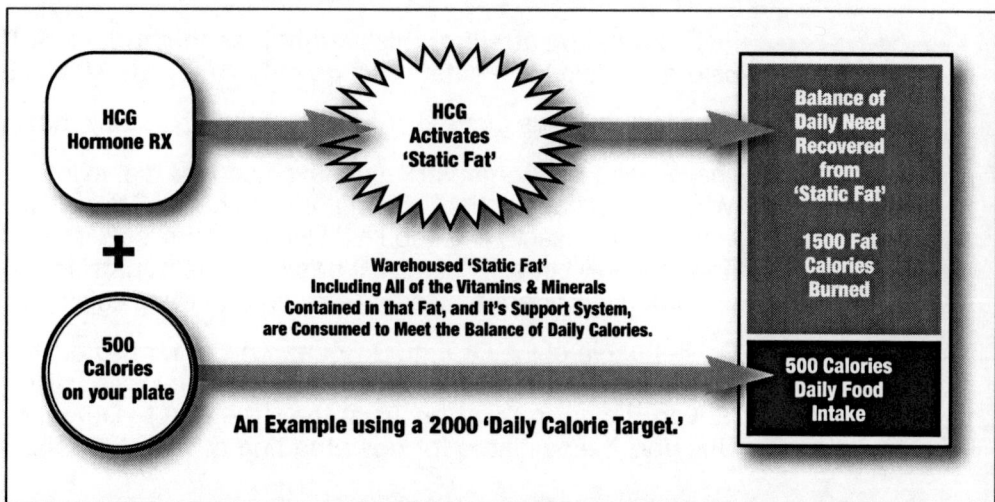

Table 3: 'Comfort & Safety Features of 'HCG Assisted' Weight Loss Method.'

HCG is the mercifully short acronym for **Human Chorionic Gonadotrophin.**

HCG is a natural human hormone and it plays **a key nutritional role** for anyone, male or female, when given in small regular doses **in concert** with the **500 Calorie** carefully structured **daily food consumption.**

As you can see in **Table 3** above, using a **2000 Calorie example,** activation by the combination of **HCG + 500 Calories,** produces several very desirable effects.

Section One: HCG + 500 Calories: BRIEF REVIEW

HCG effect on the 'static fat' allows it to be consumed by the body to meet the balance of daily Caloric needs. This takes advantage of **two natural body responses**.

First is the **low Calorie intake** of **500 Calories**, which causes your system to search for other resources. And the **second**, is the **mobilization of the stored resources** or 'static fat' you already have on board. Finding your previously stored 'static fat' which has now become 'dynamic fat' under the influence of the HCG, your system **uses that available fuel** to **satisfy the balance of your needs**.

"...mobilization of the stored resources or 'static fat' you already have on board..."

The Bottom Line.

There is no doubt that if you were **stranded on an island** and you could scrounge around and find **500 Calories** to eat... you would lose weight, and as your defense mechanisms kicked in, **you would burn your 'static fat.'** But, to say the least, you would **not** be **a happy camper!** With Dr. Simeons HCG method, I guess you could say you are tricking your body into that same 'survival' mode, **but very importantly,** at the same time, **you are releasing excess resources** to meet that need.

Appetite control is achieved with the **consumption of only 500 Calories**, without the **extreme misery and danger** of starvation. Body **weight and inches are eliminated** due to the **steady and rapid consumption of the 'warehoused fat.'**

" Appetite control is achieved with the consumption of only 500 Calories..."

Thus it is possible to leave the **good fat** untouched and **burn up the bad fat**.

However, I think you can see **why I agree 100%** with **Dr. Simeons** prescription and **Dr. Belluscio's** medical practices along with other **medical HCG experts**, when I advise you **not to proceed without an 'enlightened' doctor.**

Don't Be Afraid... But Do Choose Wisely.

Please **don't be afraid of this weight loss method**. Many thousands have gone before you and have **safely and quickly succeeded** beyond their wildest dreams.

Many critics of this method of weight loss method have **not** done their home work.

"I was skeptical at first, but now I trust it because it has been demonstrated to work, in the crucible of human experience..."

I have **done my homework** and have used the diet to lose **55 pounds in 63 days**. Many others have done the same or even better. There is **no question** in my mind that it works, exactly like good old Doc Simeons, said it would. I was **skeptical at first**, but now I trust it because it **has been demonstrated to work,** in the crucible of **human experience**, and has passed with flying colors.

Dr. Belluscio of the **Oral hCG Research Center** has done clinical testing reaffirming the validity and efficacy of the method. I recently published a paper entitled, **'Seven Reasons You Can Trust the HCG Diet to Defeat & Control Your Obesity.'** it is **available for downloading at www.HCGVictoryToolKit.com'**.

Dr. Simeons 500 Calorie Plan.

On the following pages you will find the **original 500 Calorie plan** along with some **comments** and **interpretations** of some of the common **questions and issues**, such as my take on the **HCG methods** of administration, and **immunity concerns**. **Also included are '500 Calorie Pre-made and blank 'Six Day Menu' Options' and blank forms for planning, recording and charting your progress.**

Section One:

HCG + 500 Calories: BRIEF REVIEW

*Review of
Dr. Simeons
ORIGINAL
500 calorie
diet plan.*

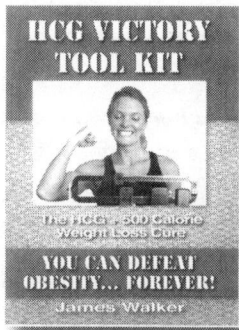

**HCG VICTORY
TOOL KIT**

The HCG + 500 Calorie
Weight Loss Cure

**YOU CAN DEFEAT
OBESITY... FOREVER!**

James Walker

*BOOK ONE:
The HCG Victory
Tool Kit ©2009*

Breakfast:

Tea or coffee in any quantity without sugar. Only one tablespoonful of milk allowed in 24 hours. Saccharin or Stevia may be used.

Lunch:

Protein: 100 grams of veal, beef, chicken breast, fresh white fish, lobster, crab, or shrimp. All visible fat must be carefully removed before cooking, and the meat must be weighed raw. It must be boiled or grilled without additional fat. Salmon, eel, tuna, herring, dried or pickled fish are not allowed.
The chicken breast must be removed from the bird.

Vegetable: One type of vegetable only to be chosen from the following: spinach, chard, chicory, beet-greens, green salad, tomatoes, celery, fennel, onions, red radishes, cucumbers, asparagus, cabbage.

Fruit: An apple, orange, or one-half grapefruit.

Breads: One breadstick (grissino) or one Melba toast.

Dinner:

Choose from the same four groups as lunch shown above BUT **avoid the same choice twice in a row.** i.e. if you have chicken for lunch then have a **different protein** choice for dinner.

Condiments & Seasonings:

The juice of one lemon daily is allowed for all purposes. Salt, pepper, vinegar, mustard powder, garlic, sweet basil, parsley, thyme, marjoram, etc., if they contain **NO SUGAR**, may be used for seasoning. **NO** oil, butter or dressing.

Drinks & Fluid Intake:

*"...the patient
should drink
about 2 liters
of these fluids
per day."*

Tea, coffee, plain water, or mineral water are the only drinks allowed, but they may be taken in any quantity and at all times. Remember **NO SUGAR.**

In fact, the patient should **drink about 2 liters** of these fluids per day. Many patients are afraid to drink so much because they fear that this may make them retain more water. This is a wrong notion as the body is more inclined to store water when the intake falls below its normal requirements.

The fruit or the breadstick may be eaten between meals instead of at lunch or dinner, but **not more than than four items**, one in each category listed, may be eaten at one meal. Remember to alternate your choices.

Section One: **HCG + 500 Calories: BRIEF REVIEW**

"This is a doctor directed treatment."

A Convenient Refresher Course

The **purpose** of this section is to to review **the essence** of the **HCG diet method**. If you want a **deeper examination** and a study of Dr. Simeons original manuscript you will find all of that in the **'HCG Victory Tool Kit.'** (Sections Two & Five)

A Closer Look at the Diet Plan.

Some of the measurements are metric, so let's look at that first.

100 grams of meat is **3.75** ounces **always weighed RAW**. Please note that is **rounded up** from the more exact 3.6 ounce equivalent of 100 grams. This is for two reasons. The first is to allow for **higher moisture content** of today's meat and poultry (up to 15%) which cooks out, and because it is an **easier measurement** to measure, on a 'garden variety' scale. It is a clear, safe and easy adjustment.

I came to this **conclusion** after studying the **primary differences** between the **proteins commonly available** today versus 40-50 years ago. This seemed like a prudent adjustment to **ensure** the **correct amount** of lean protein, a critical component of the diet. Testing by **many successful HCG dieters,** has shown that this adjustment works fine, with no negative effect. So it is **a viable option**.

Thus, **no** need to get a **fancy scale**. An **inexpensive postal scale** works just fine.

Do Not Exceed 500 Calories per Day.

Noted here are **'Four Food Groups'** for victory with **HCG + 500 Calories.**

Group One:	**Proteins**
Group Two:	**Vegetables**
Group Three:	**Fruits**
Group Four:	**Starch (in the form of Bread)**

"Yes, it is important to be as precise as possible."

Dr. Simeons did the 'Heavy Lifting.'

Fortunately for us, in the **most critical areas**, he did not leave anything to chance. We know **exactly what food options** we have and **when** to eat them.

These specific food tables by group are outlined for you in **pages 36-51** along with special **500 Calorie** pre-made **EZPlans™** using those food selections..

Remember: Rotating Your Protein Selection of is Critical.

Be careful to **rotate your choices** so you are **not eating** the **same** type **twice in a row**, for example:

   Lunch: chicken, lettuce, apple, Melba toast

   Dinner: beef, fresh spinach, grapefruit, breadstick

These **changes** in your eating plan **are important**. Another **critical point** is to stay true to the **approved choices** contained in the **'Four Food Groups.'** Dr. Simeons spent **over 40 years** working this out, just **trust it**, fly straight and **you will win**.

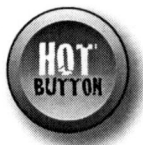

ISBN 978-0-9800641-8-6

Section One: **HCG 'Immunitiy' & 'Shots'**

"One of the most requested items is help with the preparation and selection of food options..."

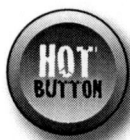

Water Water Everywhere.

Okay metrics again... a **liter** is about 34 ounces, so 2 liters a day equals **68 ounces.** Bottled water is 12 - 20 ounces, it adds up fast. **Not** getting **enough liquid** can stall your progress, so **be sure to do it right.**

Check **spices and condiments** very carefully, for any **sugar,** or **oil ingredients.**

ALL NEW Six Day 'Pre-Made EZPlans™' Save Time & Confusion.

One of the **most requested** items is help with the **preparation or selection** of food options. Once again, to make **compliance** with the stringent requirements of the good dcotor's **meticulously worked out plan,** and to keep things very **clear, simple and streamlined** I have added **a new feature.**

This **new feature** contained **in this planner** is a number of EZPlans™ designed to give you approved food group **options** in **six day** clusters. **(pages 41-51)**

'HOT BUTTON' the 'HCG Immunity Syndrome.'

"...sooner or later, interests everyone...

...the HCG Immunity Syndrome."

One other important issue, that sooner or later, **interests everyone,** is what **Dr. Simeons** refers to as the **'HCG Immunity Syndrome.'** He discusses the subject at length in his manuscript. Let's take **a closer look.**

It is **important to note** that the doctor was **never** able to **positively identify** the **underlying cause** for this so called 'immunity' reaction, but could only speculate.

In Dr. Simeons' day **this was a major issue** and a limiting **factor in the duration** of treatment. Depending on the **desired amount** of weight loss, he used a 26 or 43 day treatment or one or two 'courses' as he referred to them. Then he **would require** a **hiatus from treatment** of **at least 6 weeks,** before any resumption.

HCG in the 21st Century.

"HCG today is much more potent and you may safely repeat the twenty day course..."

The **first important point** that my personal **research** uncovered, is the indisputable **fact,** that the **HCG hormone** used today is much **more potent** and **pure,** than the **supply accessed by Dr. Simeons** some **forty years ago.**

Another conformation is the extensive research and **large number of successful cases** of obesity treated, by **Dr. Belluscio,** of the 'Oral hCG Research Center' and others world-wide, it would appear that the **underlying cause** of this phenomena **most likely** related to the **potency** and **purity of the hormone used.**

According to **current HCG medical experts,** you may safely repeat the prescribed twenty day 'course,' **up to 6 months,** or **183 days** when you add in the **three day buffer,** of non stop treatment, under the **watchful direction of your physician.** I have **personally experienced success** doing that, as have many others, all the while carrying on with their **normal lives,** including **sports activities.**

This allows you to take maximum advantage of the **'self limiting'** aspect of this protocol. Quite predictably of course, when you have **emptied** your body of it's warehoused **'abnormal fat'** you will **stop losing pounds and inches.**

That's your sign... It's **time to move on** to the next stage. That is why this planner was created, to focus more precisely, on **successful 'weight setting.'**

"... you can always return to the program anytime in the future..."

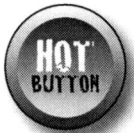

"...I like the oral methodology developed by Dr. Belluscio."

"...I most likely wouldn't have done it..."

The Bottom Line: An Even Faster Result.

So if you have **more than 20 pounds to lose, take heart,** you can usually, without a problem, keep right on going **until you reach your goal.**

In addition, if you feel you **need a 'tune-up,' you can always return to the program** anytime in the future. And as an HCG alumnus, usually with **even greater ease,** since **you know how** to manage the diet successfully. This is another reason, that this **planner** with it pages of eating options already **filled in** and plenty of supporting **forms** to help keep things **clear, simple and streamlined** was created.

Okay. Let's Talk About Needles. Ouch!

You can relax, **no shots are necessary** to successfully complete the 500 Calorie HCG assisted weight loss cure. The **'sublingual' method** is the answer I would recommend. That's doctor talk for, **'put it under your tongue and absorb it.'** It is easy to do in **minutes,** and if you are using the correct prescription should be relatively taste free.

I like the **oral methodology** developed by **Dr Belluscio.** That prescription comes as **one 20 day set** of 4 small dark bottles of the **dehydrated hormone** at a time. You simply add distilled water as directed, to **one bottle at a time.** Shake it until disolved and refrigerate it (or at least keep it cool and dark). This method assures you, that your **HCG supply is fresh** and that **consistent potency** is maintained, since you are only activating it five days at a time. A great approach.

This **oral method** is very **effective,** very **simple,** and **quick** and **non-invasive.**

Here's Why I Don't Like the 'Shots' Scene.

I must confess that if **shooting needles** into my arms and legs was the **only way** to successfully administer the HCG, **I most likely wouldn't have done it.**

Here are my Reasons:

Reason 1: We have the oral HCG formula and methodology perfected. Something that was **not available** to good old Doc Simeons. Would he have **used** the oral method as **a effective substitute** for shots? Yes. Just look at his life, and it is obvious. He was all about **ending human suffering,** he would have used the easier less painful & less invasive oral method. I have no doubt.

I **don't take issue** with those who **prefer** the shots, but **I fail to see the need.**

Reason 2: Shots are more **difficult, messier,** more **invasive** and raise a whole host of **personal hygiene** and **risks of infections** or **complications** if self administered.

Nothing to be gained from a much higher **risk** and more **difficult** administration.

Reason 3: My final reason is very personal. In 1978, at age 3 months, my youngest daughter, **Jessica,** was **severely injured** by her **DPT vaccinations.** She is totally disabled and we care for her daily in our home. So I guess you could say that shots are not very popular in our family. If you want the rest of the story, I did write a book about our experience titled, **'Growing Up with Jessica.'** (See Appendix A)

Like I said shots would have been **a 'non-starter'** for me. So there you have it.

Section One: **HCG "Starting Out Right'**

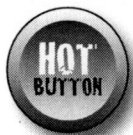

Don't Forget to 'Gorge Yourself.'

Not mentioned in Dr. Simeons short description of the **500 Calorie + HCG** diet, is an important **starting procedure** that we need to take a look at now.

One procedure, that many **people find puzzling**, is the practice of **'gorging'** on as much **fatty, high Calorie food** you can get your hands on for a minimum of two days **before you begin** the 500 Calorie part of the HCG diet. Listen to the old doctor...

"...very hard to convince of the absolute necessity of gorging for at least two days..."

"...patients who have been struggling with diets for years and know how rapidly they gain if they let themselves go are very hard to convince of the **absolute necessity of gorging for at least two days,** and yet this must he **insisted upon categorically** if the further course of treatment is to run smoothly."

This is **not optional.** Sure **you will gain a few pounds,** but doing this like the doctor said is **critical to your success.** Need I say more?

At this point you might want to take another good look at the big picture diagramed on the **'HCG Protocol Flow Chart'** on **page 14.**

Existing Health Concerns and Common Sense.

If you have any questions, **consult with your physician** or refer to the **'HCG Victory Tool Kit'** and read **Dr. Simeons cautions (pages 133-136)** in his original manuscript in **Section Five: 'Listen to the Good Doctor'** .

"...use your common sense and find an enlightened doctor that treats you with respect."

Remember this is a physician directed treatment, use your **common sense** and find an **enlightened doctor** that treats you with respect. Be a participant in your plan for health and well being, learn your options, **you are your responsibility**.

Obtain **your** complete **medical records** and keep it up to date by adding test results as they come up and anything else worthy of note. Always comes in handy.

Beneficial Side Effects Can Result.

Many of the **side effects** of HCG are **beneficial** to your health and your body. I hear about new ones all of the time, here's Dr. Simeons' list, borrowed from **'Table I'** on **page 125,** of the **'HCG Victory Tool Kit.'**

"...be a participant in your plan for health and well being, learn your options... "

Condition	Result of HCG Adminstration
Diabetes	Blood sugar drops, often possible to stop medications.
Rheumatism	Pain lessens and overall improvement within days.
Cholesterol	Improved levels 'good vs bad' and highly beneficial.
Gout	Does not occur.
Blood Pressure	Normalizes and decreases after HCG usage.
Peptic Ulcers	Subjective improvements are possible.
Psoriasis	Greatly improves, temporarily, while under treatment.
'Pregnant' male	A complete misconception. No sexual side effects

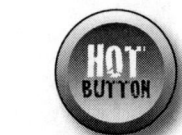

HCG + 500 CALORIES

TOOLS & HELPS

TOOLS & HELPS · HCG + 500

Loading the Chuck Wagon.

As you begin the **HCG diet + 500 Calorie step** is a good time to stock your pantry with the right things to eat and seasonings, spices and condiments that are **safe** for this critical step.

Begin by **taking inventory** of your current supplies. You may need to get out the big magnifying glass, if you have one... it's time to read that teeny tiny print **on the labels.**

CAUTION: Always Check the INGREDIENTS.

Unfortunately the originally well intentioned **'Nutrition Facts'** required on products have **become rather twisted** over the years, and can mislead, or misinform if **not carefully inspected** for hidden **sugars** and **starches** and even **incorrect** Calories.

The information on the **'Nutrition Facts'** label, can **fool you.** For instance, if the **size** of the **'suggested serving'** is **manipulated** so that the sugar content is less than 5%, then it is **not required** to be listed. However, that **sugar content**, will be **a problem** while you are **participating** in the **HCG protocol.**

"The information in the 'Nutrition Facts' label can be misleading."

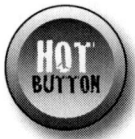

"Note the absence of sugar or starch of any kind in the ingredients listing."

"... you can easily locate what you need."

Approved Sample:

'Simply Organic Grilling Seasons.' Steak Seasoning

USDA Organic

Aha!
Here we have a seasoning that is **COMPLETELY SAFE** for you to use during your **HCG + 500 Calorie** and **NO sugar NO starch** phases.

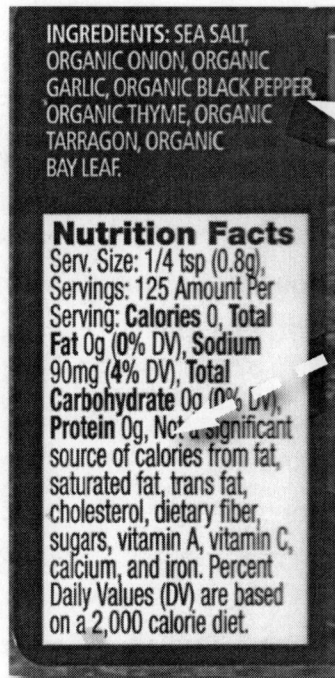

INGREDIENTS: SEA SALT, ORGANIC ONION, ORGANIC GARLIC, ORGANIC BLACK PEPPER, ORGANIC THYME, ORGANIC TARRAGON, ORGANIC BAY LEAF.

Nutrition Facts
Serv. Size: 1/4 tsp (0.8g), Servings: 125 Amount Per Serving: **Calories** 0, **Total Fat** 0g (0% DV), **Sodium** 90mg (4% DV), **Total Carbohydrate** 0g (0% DV), **Protein** 0g, Not a significant source of calories from fat, saturated fat, trans fat, cholesterol, dietary fiber, sugars, vitamin A, vitamin C, calcium, and iron. Percent Daily Values (DV) are based on a 2,000 calorie diet.

Table 4: How to Read Food Labels

Note: NO Hidden Sugars NO Hidden Starches

USDA Organic means that 95% of the ingredients used in the product are certified to be organic

Above is a label from an **'HCG safe'** seasoning product. Note t**he absence of sugar or starch** of any kind in the **ingredients** listing. That's what you are after.

Now make **a careful inspection** of the products you have on hand. You may be shocked to discover, **what is in them,** when you **look at the ingredients.**

Any sugar or starches in the **ingredients, in ANY form,** is **OFF LIMITS.**

Best to **remove those products,** at least for now, **from 'food prep' circulation.**

Section One: **HCG + 500 Calories: 'Groceries'**

Below is **a short list** of some **HCG diet safe** seasoning brands previously listed in the **'HCG Victory Tool Kit'**. You can easily locate what you need and others as well, just **carefully read all labels all the time**. Find most of them in 'health foods.'

'From the HCG Diet Victory Tool Kit'

Product	Safe Brands & Suggestions
All Natural Seasonings	Kelly's Original, Onion or Garlic
Dill Weed	Spice Islands 100% Organic
Garlic Salt	5th Season, Simply Organic
Ground Celery Salt	Tradewinds
Onion Salt	McCormick
Poultry Seasoning	Frontier Natural Products
Steak Seasoning	Simply Organic

"...a short list of some HCG Safe seasoning brands..."

Table 5: A Short List of 'HCG Safe' Seasonings

Grocery Shopping Time.

"...you may very well save on your grocery bill..."

Here's a **'Shopping List'** by the **'Four Food Groups,'** and the EZPlan™ pre-made eating plan options. Interesting fact that we have experienced, you may be spending some money for the HCG diet protocol, but **you may very well save** on your **grocery bill**. You will find that you are **eating less** overall, plus eliminating fast foods and other highly processed, highly advertised expensive products.

Food Group 1: Proteins for Victory

3.75 oz. daily.	Lean Round Steak
3.75 oz. daily.	Skinless Boneless Chicken Breasts
3.75 oz. some.	Lean fish (caution)
Optional	Chicken Eggs
Optional	Veal Round Steak

Food Group 2: Vegetables for Victory

2 Cups. daily.	Lettuces (organic pre-washed)
2 Cups. daily.	Fresh Baby Spinach Salad (organic pre-washed)

"...you are eating less overall plus eliminating 'fast foods' and other highly processed, highly advertised products."

Food Group 3: Fruits for Victory

1 Med. daily.	Apples (organic any variety)
1/2 Med. daily.	Grapefruit (red/pink/white)
1 Med. Daily	Lemon
1 Med. optional	Oranges (caution)

Food Group 4: 'Starches' for Victory

1 Stick daily.	Breadsticks (grissini)
1 Round daily.	Melba Toast

Section One: **HCG + 500 Calories: 'Groceries'**

Walk on the Wild Side.

Here are a few things that don't fit precisely in a food group, but are valuable items or **ingredients** to have in your safe eating plans. Think of them as **'wild cards.'**

Wild Card Group:

"...a few things that do fit precisely in a food group, but are valuable..."

Real Cottage Cheese	Daily allowance: 1/4 cup (58 Calories)
Real Milk	Daily allowance: 1 Tablespoon (2 Calories)
Meat Broth (organic)	Daily allowance: 1 cup (0 Calories)
Real Vinegar ('mother')	Daily allowance: 1/2 cup (1-3 Calories)
	Used for making 'Mom in a Bottle' and other dressings, condiments and recipes.

Beverages:

Coffee (organic)	Daily: No limit (8 oz. = 10 Calories)
Tea (organic)	Daily: No limit (8 oz. = 2 Calories)
Mineral Water	Daily: No limit (No Calories)
Pure Water	Daily: 68 ounces (No Calories)

SWEETENERS... If You Can't Live Without Them.

This **HCG diet** is going to allow you to **kick your sugar habit.** Here are **options**.

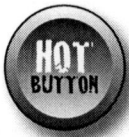

"This HCG diet is going to allow you to kick your sugar habit...

Stevia	Agave Nectar	Erythritol
Derived from the Stevia plant.The rebiana variety is best. avaliable in liquid and granulated forms.	Controversial product and to be **used with caution.** Use only pure natural Agave processed at under 118 degrees. 25% sweeter than sugar and slow absorbing.	Sugar alcohol fermented from grapes and melons. Granulated form. Fairly new on the market. So far okay.
Safe Brand Names:		**Brand Names:**
Stevia In the Raw ® **Steviva** ® **Truvia** ® **PureVia** ®	**Brand Names:** **Madhava** ® **& Wholesome** ®	**Sweet Simplicity** ® **Z Sweet** ® (also in Truvia ®)

...and as Martha might say, "That's a good thing!"

To Be 100% Avoided: Sugar by 'Any Other Name' is Still Sugar!

Barley malt	Ethyl maltol	Maltodextrin
Beet sugar	Fructose	Maltose
Brown sugar	Fruit juice	Mannitol
Buttered syrup	Fruit juice concentrate	Molasses
Cane-juice crystals	galactose	Muscovado
Cane sugar	Glucose	Panocha
Caramel	Glucose solids	Refiner's syrup
Carob syrup	Golden sugar	Rice Syrup
Corn syrup	Golden syrup	Sorbitol
Corn syrup solids	Grape sugar	Sorghum syrup
Date sugar	High-fructose corn syrup	Sucrose
Demerara Sugar	Honey	Sugar
Dextran	Invert sugar	Treacle
Dextrose	Lactose	Turbinado sugar
Diatase	Malt	Yellow sugar
Diastatic malt	Malt syrup	

Table 6: 'Sweeteners' Approach with Caution.

Section One: **HCG + 500 Calorie EZPlans**™

"...You will find... a set of 6 days worth of already prepared 500 Calorie daily food plans."

Introducing 'HCG EZPlans™' Handy Pre-Made 6 Day Food Plans.

In case you missed it, in the interest of **ease, simplicity & streamlining,** in the pages that follow are two **6 day sets,** of **prepared '500 Calorie'** daily food plans.

Putting plans together to folllow is a **stumbling block** for many HCG dieters. It is probably **impossible** to make plans that **perfectly** suit **everyone's tastes,** it is possible however, to generate **a model** plan that lays out actual options.

Most people will find these models **helpful, timesaving** and **very practical.** Lots of **time and effort** has been **devoted to that premise.** Add your **options.**

What are 'HCG EZPlans?'

They are quite simply, **a way to jump start** your HCG diet experience. They are **based on experience, medical feedback,** lots of **figuring** and **common sense.** Zeroing in on the Dr. Simeons allowed foods from the **'Four Food Groups'** as first described in **Section Four** in the **'HCG Victory Tool Kit.' (pages 55-60)**

"They all comply 100% with Dr. Simeons' prescription..."

They all **comply 100%** with **Dr. Simeons' prescription,** and are exclusively in this book, in both the **'500 Calorie + HCG'** step and the **'No Sugar or Starch' step.'**

There are **6 days** of the **500 Calorie version** in this section and also some **blank forms** if you prefer and have the time to make **your own custom plan.**

'Quite simply a way to jump start your HCG diet experience..."

Table 7: The Time Saving HCG EZPlans™

The plans shown above can be **used in any order** as long you use **odd** and **even** days and still achieve the rotation of food types indicated by Dr. Simeons. Notice that they are also **dark** and **light** for visual simplicity. Use any day in any order.

Section One: **Table 8: HCG + 500 Calories OPTIONS**

Nutritional Information on 500 Calorie Choices & Options.

Here is some **nutritional data** on the elements used in the 500 Calorie EZPlans™ Please **note** that menu elements with an **asterisk*** may be foods that trigger a weight loss problem in individual cases and are also an 'allergic' choice for some. Thus they are **not included** in the **EZPlans™**.

'Protein'	Measure or Portion	Protein (g)	Vitamins	Minerals Nutrients	Fiber (g)	Carbs (mg)	Calories
Lean Round Steak	3.75 oz.	25 g	B-12	Iron	3 grams	0	185
Skinless Chicken Breast	3.75 oz.	14 g	B & C	Calcium	0	0	85
Lean Fish*	3.75 oz.	10-30 g	B & C	Calcium	0	0	80-110
Shrimp*	3.75 oz.	25 g	-	Calcium	0	0	90-110
Crab*	3.75 oz.	18 g	C	Calcium	0	0	90-120

'Vegetables'	Portion	Protein (g)	Vitamins	Minerals Nutrients	Fiber (g)	Carbs (mg)	Calories
Average Lettuces	2 Cups	2g	C	Beta-carotene	1	4	30
Baby Spinach	1.5 Cups	1g	C & B	Calcium Beta-carotene	1	3	17
Cherry Tomatoes*	1 Cup	1g	A & C	Iron & Potassium	2	6	27
Green Onions	1 Cup	1g	C	Calcium Beta-carotene	3	2	29
Sweet Peppers	1 Cup	1g	C	Calcium Beta-carotene	3	4	29

'Fruits'	Portion	Protein (g)	Vitamins	Minerals	Fiber (g)	Carbs (mg)	Calories
Apples	1 large	0	C	Beta-carotene	3	14	75
Grapefruit	1/2 med	0	C	Calcium Beta-carotene	4	16	60
Lemons	1 med	0	C	Calcium Beta-carotene	6	5	15
Oranges*	1 med	0	C	Calcium	3	6	60
Tangerines	1 med	0	C	Calcium Beta-carotene	1	14	50

'Wild Cards'	Portion	Protein	Vitamins	Minerals	Sat Fat	Carbs (mg)	Calories
Real Cottage Cheese	1/4 Cup	7	D	Calcium Beta-carotene	2	2	58
Real Milk	1 TBSP	0	D	Calcium	2.5	1-2	2
Meat Broth	1 Cup	0	A & C	Calcium Iron	0	2	20
Real Vinegar	8 oz.	0	-	Potassium	0	1	0
Natural Yogurt	8 oz.	-	B	Calcium	8 oz.	10	100

EZPLAN™ '500 Calorie + HCG Diet Victory' EZPLAN™

DAY 1

DATE:

500 1 Record YOUR MORNING Weight:

✓ C: ITEM: SERVING:

BREAKFAST: Target 0 Calories

No breakfast is the normal approach. Drinks such as black coffee & tea, and plenty o' water is important.

LUNCH: Target 250 Calories

✓	C:	ITEM:	SERVING:
○	85	CHICKEN BRST	3.75 oz.
○	40	Green SALAD	2 Cups
○	10	Mom's DRESSING	2 oz.
○	75	APPLE Medium	WHOLE

210

DINNER: Target 250 Calories

✓	C:	ITEM:	SERVING:
○	185	Round STEAK	3.75 oz.
○	30	Spinach SALAD	1.5 Cups
○	10	Mom's DRESSING	2 oz.
○	60	GrapeFRUIT large	Half

285

495 TODAY'S Calorie TOTAL

500 Calorie Daily Plan

Optional Records & Notes:

Blood Sugar:

Blood Pressure:

Notes:

DAY 2

DATE:

500 2 Record YOUR MORNING Weight:

✓ C: ITEM: SERVING:

BREAKFAST: Target 0 Calories

No breakfast is the normal approach. Drinks such as black coffee & tea, and plenty o' water is important.

LUNCH: Target 250 Calories

✓	C:	ITEM:	SERVING:
○	85	CHICKEN BRST	3.75 oz.
○	40	Green SALAD	2 Cups
○	10	Mom's DRESSING	2 oz.
○	75	APPLE Medium	WHOLE

210

DINNER: Target 250 Calories

✓	C:	ITEM:	SERVING:
○	185	Round STEAK	3.75 oz.
○	30	Spinach SALAD	1.5 Cups
○	10	Mom's DRESSING	2 oz.
○	60	GrapeFRUIT large	Half

285

495 TODAY'S Calorie TOTAL

500 Calorie Daily Plan

Optional Records & Notes:

Blood Sugar:

Blood Pressure:

Notes:

DAY 3

DATE:

500 3 Record YOUR MORNING Weight:

✓ C: ITEM: SERVING:

BREAKFAST: Target 0 Calories

No breakfast is the normal approach. Drinks such as black coffee & tea, and plenty o' water is important.

LUNCH: Target 250 Calories

✓	C:	ITEM:	SERVING:
○	90	FISH Low Fat	3.75 oz.
○	40	Green SALAD	2 Cups
○	10	Mom's DRESSING	2 oz.
○	60	GrapeFRUIT large	Half

200

DINNER: Target 250 Calories

✓	C:	ITEM:	SERVING:
○	185	Round STEAK	3.75 oz.
○	30	Spinach SALAD	1.5 Cups
○	10	Mom's DRESSING	2 oz.
○	75	APPLE Medium	Whole

300

500 TODAY'S Calorie TOTAL

500 Calorie Daily Plan

Optional Records & Notes:

Blood Sugar:

Blood Pressure:

Notes:

Remember to Administer Your HCG as Prescribed.

EZPLAN™ '500 Calorie + HCG Diet Victory' EZPLAN™

DAY 4	DAY 5	DAY 6
500 / 4	**500 / 5**	**500 / 6**
Record YOUR MORNING Weight:	Record YOUR MORNING Weight:	Record YOUR MORNING Weight:

✓ C: ITEM: SERVING: ✓ C: ITEM: SERVING: ✓ C: ITEM: SERVING:

BREAKFAST: Target 0 Calories

Day 4	Day 5	Day 6
No breakfast is the normal approach. Drinks such as black coffee & tea, and plenty o' water is important.	No breakfast is the normal approach. Drinks such as black coffee & tea, and plenty o' water is important.	No breakfast is the normal approach. Drinks such as black coffee & tea, and plenty o' water is important.

LUNCH: Target 250 Calories

Day 4

C:	ITEM	SERVING
85	CHICKEN BRST	3.75 oz.
40	Green SALAD	2 Cups
10	Mom's DRESSING	2 oz.
75	APPLE Medium	WHOLE

210

Day 5

C:	ITEM	SERVING
85	CHICKEN BRST	3.75 oz.
40	Green SALAD	2 Cups
10	Mom's DRESSING	2 oz.
75	APPLE Medium	WHOLE

210

Day 6

C:	ITEM	SERVING
90	FISH Low Fat	3.75 oz.
40	Green SALAD	2 Cups
10	Mom's DRESSING	2 oz.
60	GrapeFRUIT large	Half

200

DINNER: Target 250 Calories

Day 4

C:	ITEM	SERVING
185	Round STEAK	3.75 oz.
30	Spinach SALAD	1.5 Cups
10	Mom's DRESSING	2 oz.
60	GrapeFRUIT large	Half

285

Day 5

C:	ITEM	SERVING
185	Round STEAK	3.75 oz.
30	Spinach SALAD	1.5 Cups
10	Mom's DRESSING	2 oz.
60	GrapeFRUIT large	Half

285

Day 6

C:	ITEM	SERVING
185	Round STEAK	3.75 oz.
30	Spinach SALAD	1.5 Cups
10	Mom's DRESSING	2 oz.
75	APPLE Medium	Whole

300

495 TODAY'S Calorie TOTAL	495 TODAY'S Calorie TOTAL	500 TODAY'S Calorie TOTAL

500 Calorie Daily Plan
Optional Records & Notes:

Blood Sugar:

Blood Pressure:

Notes:

500 Calorie Daily Plan
Optional Records & Notes:

Blood Sugar:

Blood Pressure:

Notes:

500 Calorie Daily Plan
Optional Records & Notes:

Blood Sugar:

Blood Pressure:

Notes:

Remember to Administer Your HCG as Prescribed.

EZPLAN™ '500 Calorie + HCG Diet Victory'   EZPLAN™

DATE:	**DATE:**	**DATE:**

500	Record YOUR MORNING Weight:	500	Record YOUR MORNING Weight:	500	Record YOUR MORNING Weight:

☑ C: ITEM: SERVING: ☑ C: ITEM: SERVING: ☑ C: ITEM: SERVING:

BREAKFAST: Target 0 Calories   BREAKFAST: Target 0 Calories   BREAKFAST: Target 0 Calories

No breakfast is the normal approach. Drinks such as black coffee & tea, and plenty o' water is important.

No breakfast is the normal approach. Drinks such as black coffee & tea, and plenty o' water is important.

No breakfast is the normal approach. Drinks such as black coffee & tea, and plenty o' water is important.

LUNCH: Target 250 Calories   LUNCH: Target 250 Calories   LUNCH: Target 250 Calories

DINNER: Target 250 Calories   DINNER: Target 250 Calories   DINNER: Target 250 Calories

TODAY'S Calorie TOTAL   **TODAY'S Calorie TOTAL**   **TODAY'S Calorie TOTAL**

500 Calorie Daily Plan
Optional Records & Notes:

Blood Sugar:

Blood Pressure:

Notes:

500 Calorie Daily Plan
Optional Records & Notes:

Blood Sugar:

Blood Pressure:

Notes:

500 Calorie Daily Plan
Optional Records & Notes:

Blood Sugar:

Blood Pressure:

Notes:

Remember to Administer Your HCG as Prescribed.

EZPLAN™ '500 Calorie + HCG Diet Victory'   EZPLAN™

DATE:	DATE:	DATE:
500 / Record YOUR MORNING Weight:	500 / Record YOUR MORNING Weight:	500 / Record YOUR MORNING Weight:

✓ C: ITEM: SERVING: ✓ C: ITEM: SERVING: ✓ C: ITEM: SERVING:

BREAKFAST: Target 0 Calories

No breakfast is the normal approach. Drinks such as black coffee & tea, and plenty o' water is important.

No breakfast is the normal approach. Drinks such as black coffee & tea, and plenty o' water is important.

No breakfast is the normal approach. Drinks such as black coffee & tea, and plenty o' water is important.

LUNCH: Target 250 Calories

○ _____
○ _____
○ _____
○ _____

_____

DINNER: Target 250 Calories

○ _____
○ _____
○ _____
○ _____

_____

TODAY'S Calorie TOTAL

---

500 Calorie Daily Plan

Optional Records & Notes:

Blood Sugar:

Blood Pressure:

Notes:

Remember to Administer Your HCG as Prescribed.

EZPLAN™ '500 Calorie + HCG Diet Victory' EZPLAN™

DATE: | **DATE:** | **DATE:**

| 500 | Record YOUR MORNING Weight: | 500 | Record YOUR MORNING Weight: | 500 | Record YOUR MORNING Weight: |

☑ C: ITEM: SERVING: | ☑ C: ITEM: SERVING: | ☑ C: ITEM: SERVING:

BREAKFAST: Target 0 Calories

No breakfast is the normal approach. Drinks such as black coffee & tea, and plenty o' water is important.

No breakfast is the normal approach. Drinks such as black coffee & tea, and plenty o' water is important.

No breakfast is the normal approach. Drinks such as black coffee & tea, and plenty o' water is important.

LUNCH: Target 250 Calories

○ ____ _____ _____
○ ____ _____ _____
○ ____ _____ _____
○ ____ _____ _____

_____

DINNER: Target 250 Calories

○ ____ _____ _____
○ ____ _____ _____
○ ____ _____ _____
○ ____ _____ _____

_____

| | TODAY'S Calorie TOTAL | | TODAY'S Calorie TOTAL | | TODAY'S Calorie TOTAL |

500 Calorie Daily Plan

Optional Records & Notes:

Blood Sugar:

Blood Pressure:

Notes:

Remember to Administer Your HCG as Prescribed.

EZPLAN™ '500 Calorie + HCG Diet Victory' EZPLAN™

DATE:	DATE:	DATE:
500 Record YOUR MORNING Weight:	**500** Record YOUR MORNING Weight:	**500** Record YOUR MORNING Weight:

✓ C: ITEM: SERVING: ✓ C: ITEM: SERVING: ✓ C: ITEM: SERVING:

BREAKFAST: Target 0 Calories

No breakfast is the normal approach. Drinks such as black coffee & tea, and plenty o' water is important.

No breakfast is the normal approach. Drinks such as black coffee & tea, and plenty o' water is important.

No breakfast is the normal approach. Drinks such as black coffee & tea, and plenty o' water is important.

LUNCH: Target 250 Calories

DINNER: Target 250 Calories

TODAY'S Calorie TOTAL

TODAY'S Calorie TOTAL

TODAY'S Calorie TOTAL

500 Calorie Daily Plan
Optional Records & Notes:

Blood Sugar:

Blood Pressure:

Notes:

500 Calorie Daily Plan
Optional Records & Notes:

Blood Sugar:

Blood Pressure:

Notes:

500 Calorie Daily Plan
Optional Records & Notes:

Blood Sugar:

Blood Pressure:

Notes:

Remember to Administer Your HCG as Prescribed.

Section Two:

'Weight Setting'

> "We are what we
> repeatedly do.
> Excellence, then,
> is not an act
> but a habit"
>
> *Aristotle*

Defeat OBESITY...Forever!

The HCG Assisted 500 Calorie Weight Loss Cure

Section Two:

No 'Sugar or Starch' Zone: BRIEF OVERVIEW

**STEP 4
No Sugar
No Starch
to Set
Weight**

*"...succeed in
setting your
bodies new
'weight set point,
it is very
important..."*

*"All NEW
'Weight &
Calorie
Worksheet..."*

*"All NEW
time saving
EZPlans™
for
1200 to 2600
Calorie targets..."*

Weight Setting Step: It's Only 3 Weeks!

Now that you have lost all that weight, your next step is to **succeed** in setting your bodies **new 'weight set point.'** It is VERY IMPORTANT that you **avoid sugars & starches** of any kind, in any quantity. And also consume the correct amount of Calories for your final HCG day weight. **Review the Tables on pages 14 and 20.**

Time Saving TOOLS for 'Calorie Targets' & 'Menu Plans'

In this section you will find:

- **All NEW 'Weight Setting Worksheets'**
- **Exclusive** Dr. Simeons **safe, 'SEE-Food' Diet Tables'** with **'Food Options & Alternatives'**
- **NEW time saving pre-made 'EZPlans.'**™ for **1200 to 2600 Calorie targets** in **100 Calorie** increments. Provided in pre-made **6 day models PLUS** Bonus **blank forms** for **customization**
- **Tips & Tricks: 'Adapting to Family Meal Planning'**
- **Guide for Estimating Measurements on the Fly.**

'Fill'er Up... with Calories.

The most **common challenge** in the **No Sugar/NO Starch phase** is to **eat enough** Calories! The EZPlan™ menu models were developed to help with this issue, by providing a precise workable plan, with a minimum of effort.

As the **HCG effect leaves** your body, you **will not** physically be able to continue on eating **500 Calories** a day... don't kid yourself, and don't let your over enthusiasm, throw you off course.

Starvation Does Not Work... Here's What Does!

Remember **your body's system** will **try to go back** to the weight **you were** before treatment. You need to have a **general idea** of the correct range of **daily Calories required** for your final body weight. Then you are ready for 'weight setting.'

Okay. Here's the Drill.

You don't have to memorize this but here is an outline of the key points.

(1) Your final daily weight on your final HCG day is your new weight.

(2) Use 'Weight Setting Worksheet' on page 57-61 to get your 'Calorie Target.'

(3) Choose the pre-made EZplan™ that meets your 'Calorie Target.'

(4) Follow the EZplan™ weighing daily and recording your weight.

(5) If you exceed the 2 pound limit take corrective actions.

If you are **over the 2 pound limit** even a **tenth** of a pound, you need a **course correction**. Begin by reviewing the protocol **flow chart** on **page 14**. Complete instructions for the proper use of a 'steak day' is in Appendix C: Troubleshooting'

Section Two: No 'Sugar or Starch' Zone: BRIEF OVERVIEW

NO SUGAR or SUGAR ADDITIVES or STARCHS.

You don't have to hit your Calories exactly, remember it is **a target** to shoot for. The **only number** you must be **precise** with, is your **morning weight**. Be **consistent** with time of day, what you're wearing, the scale (when traveling, take it). Remember... **immediate action** is required. Do the **'steak day'** that very day.

"If you are over the 2 pound limit even a tenth of a pound, you need a course correction."

Do the 'Weight Setting Worksheet' to Find Your Calorie Targets.

First you need to determine your **correct daily Calorie** consumption **targets.**

Your **enlightened physician** can help as well, but on **the following page** is a **simple method**, based on some of the most up to date information.

Remember **you must eat enough** and keep the **protein up** and the **balance** that you had on the 500 Calorie menu. **A quick review: 40%** protein, **30%** fruits, **30%** vegetables, seems to be **a very successful ratio** and seems to work for most all 'metabolic types.' After studying Dr. Simeons writings, that does not surprise me.

We will cover **more about** what I like to call **'metabolic blueprints'** in **Section Three: 'Returning to Earth.'** It is a fascinating topic and one that I feel dovetails and **correlates very well** with Dr. Simeons fine work.

Getting the Most from the 1200 to 2600 Calorie EZPlans™

"The EZPlans™ cover 1200 to 2600 Calories in 100 Calorie increments..."

These plans, as I have said earlier, cannot please everyone, but the **intention** is to present **a working model** to help guide you and to help you visualize how to make this step work, with the minimum amount of time and fuss. You can concentrate on just staying on the plan for the next **three weeks**. You are almost there!

Some Suggested Way to Use & Adapt the EZPlans™

- Use the EZPlans™ Exactly as Written.

- Repeat Your Favorite Day or Use the 7th Day as a 'Steak or Apple Day'

- Mix or Match using any combination of Odd and Even Days

- Modify to Suite You Using the 'See-Food' Diet Charts.

- Write Your Own Plan from Scratch Using The EZplans™ as a Guide.

"...you must eat enough and keep the protein up..."

You can easily **develop a custom eating plan** using the **blank forms** included for that purpose. Some dieters have success by **simply eliminating** or substituting any food type that they **overreact** to, such as, oranges, tomatoes or seafood. Check the **'SEE-FOOD' diet charts** on **pages 65-68** for optional choices.

Another move with **a persistent** weight gain problem is to **drop 100 Calories** from your daily Calorie plan. This is easy to accomplish since the **EZPlans™** cover **1200 to 2600** Caories in **100 Calorie increments** to faciltate **any fine tuning**.

As highlighted above, these are 6 day plans, so that you can use **the 7th day as you wish** Just string 21 days together, watch your daily weight, and you are done!

Section Two: **Weight Setting WORKSHEET**

An Adventure in Weight & Calorie Goals.

One of the **first things** you need is **a target** to shoot for, or you probably **won't hit anything**. At this step you are shooting to **keep your weight within 2 lbs.** of your **'final' weight**, which is taken on the **last day** of your '500 Calorie + HCG' step. In the **'HCG Victory Tool Kit'** on pages **180-181** are some simple charts and estimates **that will work just fine** if you **like that option**. They have worked for thousands before you.

In this planner you have a selection of **pre-made eating options** that are in **100 calorie increments**. Thinking, that perhaps you might like to have a more precise option for calculating your **post HCG calorie targets**, I researched it and found a more scientific method (think egghead) way to **map your targets**.

The result is the **worksheet below,** leaving out all of the technical big words. It does work very well and may **satisfy** your inner nerd yearnings. It is **simple** and **fun** and a gives you **a good place to start**.

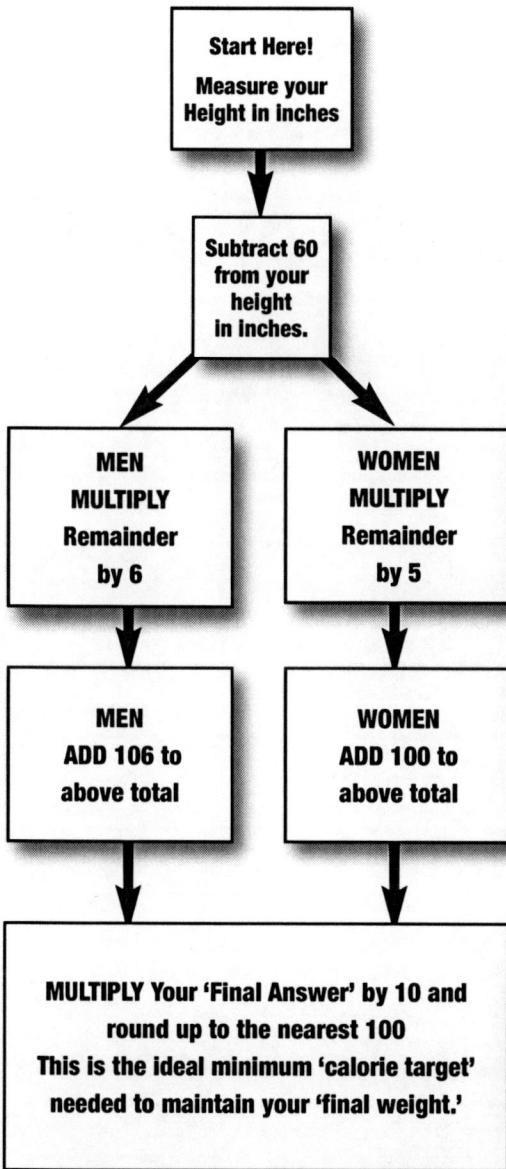

Start Here! Measure your Height in inches	Height in INCHES _____
↓	SUBTRACT 60 _____
Subtract 60 from your height in inches.	REMAINDER is _____

MEN:

Remainder X **6** _____

ADD **106** _____

Total X **10** _____

Round your ANSWER UP to **nearest 100**. _____

MEN MULTIPLY Remainder by 6	**WOMEN** MULTIPLY Remainder by 5

WOMEN:

Remainder X **5** _____

ADD **100** _____

Total X **10** _____

Round your ANSWER UP to **nearest 100.**

MEN ADD 106 to above total	**WOMEN** ADD 100 to above total

Please Note: This number represents your MINIMUM daily 'Calorie target' to keep your body functioning. An AVERAGE person with AVERAGE activity should be able to safely add 20% to the above 'final answer' to determine a safe daily 'Calorie Target.'

MULTIPLY Your 'Final Answer' by 10 and round up to the nearest 100 This is the ideal minimum 'calorie target' needed to maintain your 'final weight.'

Your 'Final Answer' _____

Always round up to the nearest 100 Calories.

Table 9: 'Calorie Targets' Flow Chart

Section Two: Weight Setting WORKSHEET

An Adventure in Weight & Calorie Goals.

One of the **first things** you need is **a target** to shoot for, or you probably **won't hit anything**. At this step you are shooting to **keep your weight within 2 lbs.** of your 'final' weight, which is taken on the **last day** of your '500 Calorie + HCG' step. In the **'HCG Victory Tool Kit'** on pages **180-181** are some simple charts and estimates **that will work just fine** if you **like that option**. They have worked for thousands before you.

In this planner you have a selection of **pre-made eating options** that are in **100 calorie increments**. Thinking, that perhaps you might like to have a more precise option for calculating your **post HCG calorie targets**, I researched it and found a more scientific method (think egghead) way to **map your targets**.

The result is the **worksheet below,** leaving out all of the technical big words. It does work very well and may **satisfy** your inner nerd yearnings. It is **simple** and **fun** and a gives you **a good place to start**.

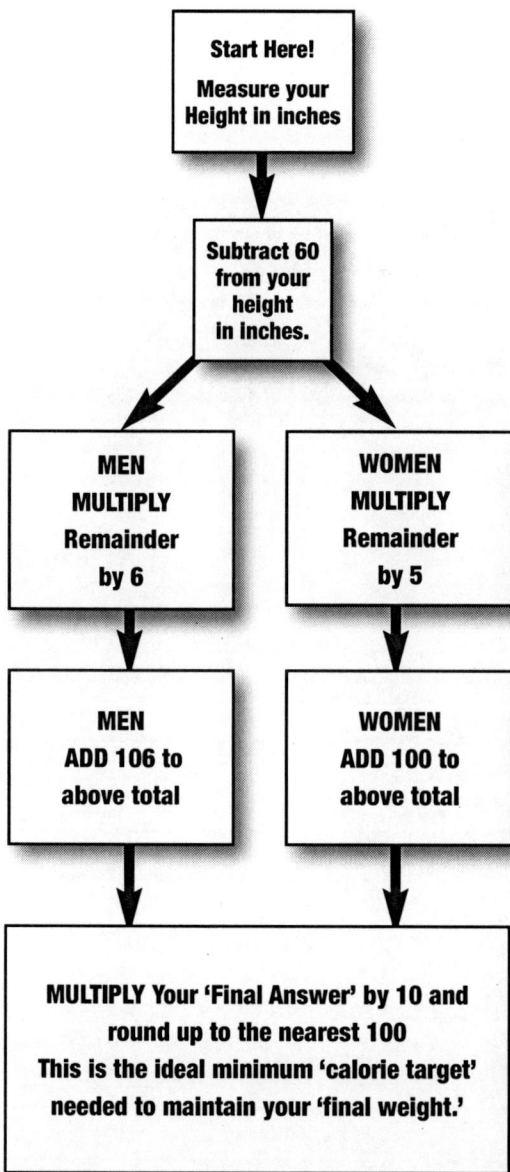

<table>
<tr><td>

Start Here!

Measure your Height in inches

↓

Subtract 60 from your height in inches.

↙ ↘

MEN MULTIPLY Remainder by 6	WOMEN MULTIPLY Remainder by 5
↓	↓
MEN ADD 106 to above total	WOMEN ADD 100 to above total

↓

MULTIPLY Your 'Final Answer' by 10 and round up to the nearest 100
This is the ideal minimum 'calorie target' needed to maintain your 'final weight.'

</td><td>

Height in INCHES   _____

SUBTRACT 60   _____

REMAINDER is   _____

MEN:

Remainder X **6**   _____

ADD **106**   _____

Total X **10**   _____

Round your ANSWER UP
to **nearest 100.**   _____

WOMEN:

Remainder X **5**   _____

ADD **100**   _____

Total X **10**   _____

Round your ANSWER UP to **nearest 100.**

Your 'Final Answer'   _____

Please Note: This number represents your MINIMUM daily 'Calorie target' to keep your body functioning. An AVERAGE person with AVERAGE activity should be able to safely add 20% to the above 'final answer' to determine a safe daily 'Calorie Target.'

Always round up to the nearest 100 Calories.

</td></tr>
</table>

Table 9: 'Calorie Targets' Flow Chart

Section Two:	Weight Setting WORKSHEET

An Adventure in Weight & Calorie Goals.

One of the **first things** you need is **a target** to shoot for, or you probably **won't hit anything**. At this step you are shooting to **keep your weight within 2 lbs.** of your 'final' weight, which is taken on the **last day** of your '500 Calorie + HCG' step. In the **'HCG Victory Tool Kit'** on pages **180-181** are some simple charts and estimates **that will work just fine** if you **like that option**. They have worked for thousands before you.

In this planner you have a selection of **pre-made eating options** that are in **100 calorie increments**. Thinking, that perhaps you might like to have a more precise option for calculating your **post HCG calorie targets**, I researched it and found a more scientific method (think egghead) way to **map your targets**.

The result is the **worksheet below,** leaving out all of the technical big words. It does work very well and may **satisfy** your inner nerd yearnings. It is **simple** and **fun** and a gives you **a good place to start**.

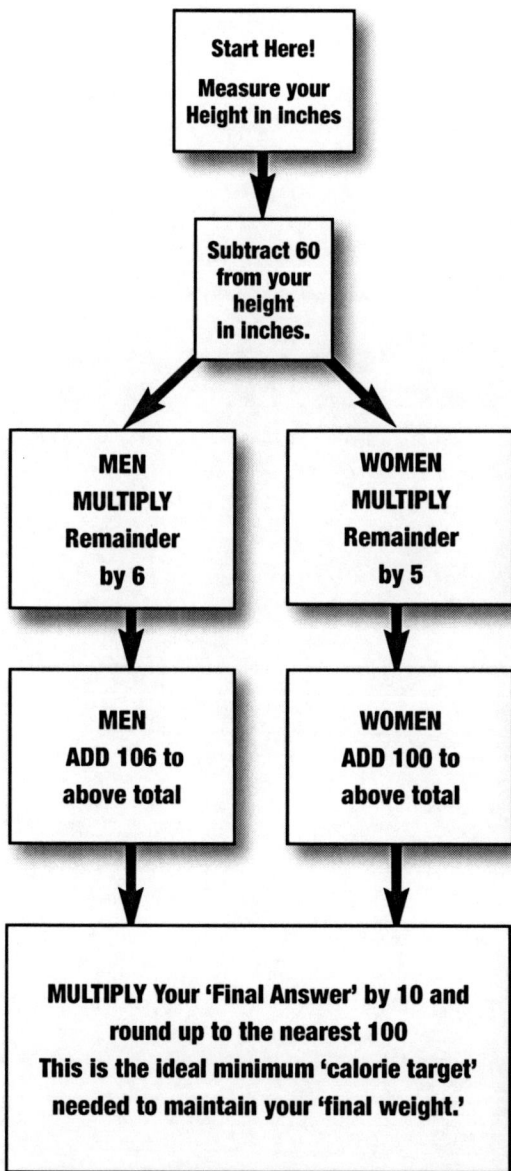

Height in INCHES _____

SUBTRACT 60 _____

REMAINDER is _____

MEN:

Remainder X **6** _____

ADD **106** _____

Total X **10** _____

Round your ANSWER UP
to **nearest 100.** _____

WOMEN:

Remainder X **5** _____

ADD **100** _____

Total X **10** _____

Round your ANSWER UP to **nearest 100.**

Your 'Final Answer' _____

Please Note: This number represents your MINIMUM daily 'Calorie target' to keep your body functioning. An AVERAGE person with AVERAGE activity should be able to safely add 20% to the above 'final answer' to determine a safe daily 'Calorie Target.'

Always round up to the nearest 100 Calories.

Start Here!
Measure your Height in inches

Subtract 60 from your height in inches.

MEN MULTIPLY Remainder by 6

WOMEN MULTIPLY Remainder by 5

MEN ADD 106 to above total

WOMEN ADD 100 to above total

MULTIPLY Your 'Final Answer' by 10 and round up to the nearest 100
This is the ideal minimum 'calorie target' needed to maintain your 'final weight.'

Table 9: 'Calorie Targets' Flow Chart

©HCGDietVictoryPlanner.com

ISBN 978-0-9800641-8-6

NO SUGAR OR STARCH

FOUR FOOD GROUPS

NO SUGAR NO STARCH FOODS

Section Two: No 'Sugar or Starch' 'SEE-FOOD' Options.

The Full Set of OPTIONS: Don't SEE IT... Don't Eat it...that's the PLAN!

You should have your daily **'Calorie target'** set and now be ready to **start** using the appropriate **'No Sugar or Starch' EZPlan™**. For reference, here are the **proper food groups** from the ' **HCG Victory Tool Kit,'** just in case you want to do some **OPTIONAL customization** to the EZPlans™.

Select the correct **daily target count shown** at the top of the **EZplan™**. They run from 1200 to 2600.

The **'Menu OPTIONS' listed on the next few pages,** are in alphabetical order by category and within each category. Carbs are noted, sugar is not, because any 'natural' sugar that is an integral part of the food selections originally approved by Dr. Simeons, can normally be consumed in this step, without a problem. It's just the **added sugars** or **starchy foods** that are **prohibited** during the next three weeks.

It's Okay to Customize Within Limits.

Using the **EZPlans™** that begin on **page 71**, and all of the ways you can use them, including using the blank forms on **pages 131-139**, along with the options provided here, you are all set for success.

DRINKS: 3 Week-No Sugar/Starch OPTIONS

Water, Water Everywhere...

Okay this is a good place to start. Getting **plenty of liquids** is, as always, important for your health. Not a lot of Calories to worry about if you follow the chart. No sugars or dairy products added. **68 ounces**.

Description	Serving Size	Calories	Protein	Fiber	Carbs	Notes:
COFFEE	8 oz	0	0	0	0	**Black**
LEMON JUICE, Fresh	4 oz	30	0	0	10	
LIME JUICE, Fresh	8 oz	30	1	0	10	
TOMATO JUICE	4 oz	20	1	0	5	
V-8 JUICE	4 oz	25	1	1	5	
WATER, Pure	8 oz	0	0	0	0	**No Limit**

DAIRY: 3 Week-No Sugar/Starch OPTIONS

Making the Most with the Least.

You can use these two **Dairy based products** to augment your recipes and add variety and some safe Calories to your daily plan. Remember to keep the **variety and rotation** going.

Note that the pudding choice here may contain **aspartame** as a sweetener. You will have to decide. We are only talking about **a three week period** and the pudding does fill in the 'dessert' slot. Helps fill the 'chocolate' void and is **fat free** and **low calorie**. There are **some reasonable trade-offs** there.

Description	Serving Size	Calories	Protein	Fat	Sat Fat	Notes:
COTTAGE CHEESE, Small Curd	4 TBSP	60	0	0	0	**Real**
PUDDING, Fat Free-Sugar Free	4 oz	70	0	0	0	**Milk**

FRUITS: 3 Week-No Sugar/Starch OPTIONS

Expanding Your Fruit Palette.

Now you can start **adding more fruits** to your meals. Add new flavors and great eye appeal. A safe way to bulk up your Calories. Keep good **records** and watch the **balance** and **rotation**.

Description	Serving Size	Calories	Protein	Fiber	Carbs	Notes:
APPLES	1 med.	75	0	3	19	Organic
APPLESAUCE-Unsweetened	3 oz	35	0	1	11	Organic
BLACKBERRIES	1 Cup	55	0	2	14	Raw
BLUEBERRIES	1 Cup	40	1	4	11	Raw
CRANBERRIES, Dried	2 Tbsp	44	0	1	12	No sugar
GRAPEFRUIT	1/2 med	60	1	4	14	No sugar
RASPBERRIES	1 Cup	50	1	3	13	Raw
STRAWBERRIES	1 Cup	68	1	5	16	Raw
NECTARINES	1 med	70	1	1	16	Organic
PEACHES	1 med	38	1	1	9	Organic
PLUMS	1 med	30	0	2	8	Organic
TANGERINES	1 med	50	1	2	14	Organic

MEAT & EGGS: 3 Week-No Sugar/Starch OPTIONS

Add Lean Pork & Even Bacon to Your Menu OPTIONS.

Continue to trim fat and weigh raw, keeping in mind your protein balance and increased Caloric needs.

Description	Serving Size	Calories	Protein	Fiber	Carbs	Notes:
EGGS, Poached	1 Large	76	6	0	0	No OIL
BACON	1 slice	34	2	0	0	
BEEF, Lean Steak	3.75 oz	185	25	0	0	
BEEF, Roast	1 oz	170	24	0	0	
CHICKEN, Breast-Broiled/Baked	3.75 oz	70	14	2	2	Skinless
FISH, Low Fat-Baked/Broiled	3.75 oz	90	30	0	0	
PORK CHOPS, Lean Center Cut	3.75 oz	150	20	0	0	Trimmed
TURKEY/CHICKEN, Hot Dog	1 dog	100	6	0	1	
SHRIMP, broiled/barbequed	3.75 oz	100	20	0	0	No Sauce

VEGETABLE TALES: 3 Week-No Sugar/Starch OPTIONS

A Great Supporting Cast

Not a lot of Calories here. So you may find it **challenging** to keep your veggies up in the 30% range of your daily plan. The good news is you can eat these like crazy. Keep **good records**, because as previously mentioned, tomatoes* can be a problem for some people. I was one of those. This gives you a lot **more vegetables** for your rotation. Also you can start mixing them in your salads and meals.

Description	Serving Size	Calories	Protein	Fiber	Carbs	Notes:
ALFALFA SPROUTS	1/2 Cup	5	1	1	1	Salad
ASPARAGUS	4 oz	25	3	2	0	Steamed
BROCCOLI	1 Cup	44	5	5	6	Steamed
BRUSSEL SPROUTS	1 Cup	38	3	3	8	Steamed
CABBAGE	4 oz	28	1	1	6	Salad
CARROTS, Cooked or Raw	1/2 Cup	30	1	2	6	
CELERY	1 Cup	18	1	2	4	Raw
CHERRY TOMATOES*	1 Cup	28	1	2	3	Salad
CUCUMBERS, 'Larry size'	1 Cup	16	1	1	3	Salad
EGGPLANT	1 Cup	35	1	2	9	
GREEN BEANS, Cooked	1 Cup	38	2	4	8	
LETTUCE, All Varieties	1 Cup	20	2	2	0	Salad
MUSHROOMS	4 med	15	2	0	3	Salad
ONIONS, Green RAW	1 Cup	25	1	1	1	Chopped
ONIONS, Red, Yellow, White	1 Cup	30	1	1	7	Trimmed
PEPPERS, Hot Chili-red/green	1 med	15	1	1	3	Salad
PEPPERS, Bell-All Colors	1 Cup	30	1	1	7	Salad
RADISHES, Raw	1 Cup	30	1	1	1	Salad
SPINACH, Raw	1 Cup	12	1	0	0	Salad
SPINACH, COOKED	1 Cup	42	5	0	0	

Yes, You Can... Set Up Your Own Plan.

Remember you can use the **EZPlans**™ in a variety of ways to achieve success. **Note:** In the **EZPlan**™ section you will find **premade & blank forms** if you prefer to develop your own custom plans. All of the forms contain 6 days not seven. This is to allow you the freedom to repeat your favorite day, or to create your own seventh day using your food favorites or do a 'steak or apple day.' Keep **good records** and keep **making the necessary adjustments & course corrections**. A good approach is to **do a great one week plan** and just repeat it 3 times to complete your **21 days**. When you have finished you are ready to **move on to 'Step 5.'**

Section Two: **Tips & Tricks: Families & Portion Management**

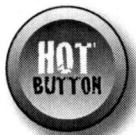

A Simple Method for Including Members of Your Family

Take a **closer look** at the **EZPlans™** and you will notice that they are based on 'food elements' as opposed to 'food recipes.' This is helpful when including non-dieting famly members in your meal plans. An especially valuable concept to grasp if you are the primary 'care giver,' when it comes to family meal planning and preparation.

Family Support: A Critical Element of Your HCG Diet Victory.

They can make you or break you. In fact **Dr. Simeons wisely met** with the **'food preparer'** in the family, because he knew, they needed to be on the same page for maximum success to follow. It was true then and it is true now.

Using **your new found skill** at weighing and estimating your food choices you can take a couple of approaches to **fit your family in** and... avoid the mutiny.

Healthier & Delicious Multiple Choices.

The **EZPlans™** give you a wide range of daily plans from 1200 to 2600 Calories, each **using multiples of the basic unit**. For instance the protein is in multples of 3.75 oz. So you can continue to process store and prepare, in the same way you have become accustomed. Use the '**Weight Setting Worksheets**' (p 57-61) if needed.

Using the healthy **'food elements'** and optional choices provided, it is then possible to prepare a delicious variety of recipes. The third book in this series is **a recipe book** that continues in that modular theme. As someone once said, **"...bon appétité! "**

"Dr. Simeons wisely met with the 'food preparer' in the family..."

"...a couple of approaches to fit your family in and... avoid the mutiny"

"...easily learn portion estimating on the fly."

Guides for Measuring & Estimating PORTIONS.

If you want to carry a set of measuring cups, you certainly could, but for most of us, it's just not practical. Here is **a list of sizes** and some **familiar objects** to help you **easily learn portion estimating** on the fly. You may find this very helpful.

Just HOW BIG is...	...COMPARED TO these familiar items.
1 Teaspoon (tsp)	Same size as the TIP of your INDEX FINGER.
1 Tablespoon (TBSP)	Same size as the TOP half of your THUMB.
1/2 Cup	Half the Size of your balled FIST is a good guide.
1 Cup	The Size of your balled FIST is a good guide.
1 Medium Fruit	Same size as a BASEBALL.
1 oz. Cheese	Same size as your THUMB is a good guide.
3-4 oz. of MEAT	Same size as a deck of cards
5-6 oz. of MEAT	Same size as TWO decks of cards

Section Two: No 'Sugar or Starch' EZPlans™

NO SUGAR OR STARCH

TIME SAVING EZPLANS™

TIME SAVING EZPLANS

'NO Sugar & Starch Diet Victory' EZPLAN™   1200 Calories

Day 1

DATE:

1200 · 1 Record YOUR MORNING Weight:

✓	C:	ITEM:	SERVING:
		BREAKFAST	
○	76	POACHED EGG	1 Large
○	34	BACON Slice	1
○	70	Applesauce	6 oz.
○	50	V8 Juice	8 oz.
○	60	Grapefruit	1/2
	290	Breakfast Total	
		Snack 1	
○	60	Cottage Cheese	4 TBSP
○	40	BlueBerries	1 Cup
	100	Snack 1 Total	
		Lunch	
○	170	CHICKEN BRST (2)	7.5 oz.
○	40	Green SALAD	2 Cups
○	10	Mom's DRESSING	2 oz.
○	75	Apple Sliced	1 med
	295	Lunch Total	
		Snack 2	
○	50	Pudding (NS)	4 oz.
○	68	Strawberries (NS)	1 Cup
	118	Snack 2 Total	
		Dinner	
○	185	Round STEAK	3.75 oz.
○	30	Spinach SALAD	1.5 Cups
○	10	Mom's DRESSING	2 oz.
○	70	Apple Sauce (NS)	6 oz.
	295	Dinner Total	
		Snack 3	
○	50	Pudding (NS)	4 oz.
○	40	BlueBerries	1 Cup
	90	Snack 3 Total	

1208 TODAY'S Calorie TOTAL

Day 2

DATE:

1200 · 2 Record YOUR MORNING Weight:

✓	C:	ITEM:	SERVING:
		BREAKFAST	
○	76	POACHED EGG	1 Large
○	100	Chicken Sausage	1
○	70	Applesauce*	6 oz.
○	20	Tomato Juice	4 oz.
○	60	Grapefruit	1/2
	326	Breakfast Total	
		Snack 1	
○	50	Pudding (NS)	4 oz.
○	40	BlueBerries	1 Cup
	90	Snack 1 Total	
		Lunch	
○	185	Round STEAK	3.75 oz.
○	40	Spinach SALAD	2 Cups
○	10	Mom's DRESSING	2 oz.
○	75	Apple Sliced	1 med
	310	Lunch Total	
		Snack 2	
○	60	Cottage Cheese	4 TBSP
○	68	Strawberries (NS)	1 Cups
	128	Snack 2 Total	
		Dinner	
○	170	CHICKEN BRST	7.5 oz.
○	30	Green SALAD	1.5 Cups
○	10	Mom's DRESSING	2 oz.
○	70	Apple Fresh Sliced	1 med
	280	Dinner Total	
		Snack 3	
○	50	Pudding (NS)	7.5 oz.
○	28	Blackberries (NS)	1/2 Cup
	78	Snack 2 Total	

1232 TODAY'S Calorie TOTAL

Day 3

DATE:

1200 · 3 Record YOUR MORNING Weight:

✓	C:	ITEM:	SERVING:
		BREAKFAST	
○	152	POACHED EGGS	2 Large
○	40	BlueBerries	1 Cup
○	70	Applesauce*	6 oz.
○	50	V8 Juice	8 oz.
○	34	Strawberries	1/2 Cup
	346	Breakfast Total	
		Snack 1	
○	50	Raspberries	1 Cup
○	50	Pudding (NS)	4 oz.
	100	Snack 1 Total	
		Lunch	
○	170	CHICKEN BRST (2)	7.5 oz.
○	40	Green SALAD	2 Cups
○	10	Mom's DRESSING	2 oz.
○	68	Strawberries (NS)	1 Cup
	288	Lunch Total	
		Snack 2	
○	60	Cottage Cheese	4 TBSP
○	55	Blackberries (NS)	1 Cup
	115	Snack 2 Total	
		Dinner	
○	185	Round STEAK	3.75 oz.
○	30	Green SALAD	1.5 Cups
○	10	Mom's DRESSING	2 oz.
○	38	Peach Sliced	1 med
	263	Dinner Total	
		Snack 3	
○	50	Pudding (NS)	1/2 Large
○	40	BlueBerries	1 Cup
	90	Snack 2 Total	

1202 TODAY'S Calorie TOTAL

'NO Sugar & Starch Diet Victory' EZPLAN™ | 1200 Calories

DAY 4 — 1200

DATE:

Record YOUR MORNING Weight:

✓	C:	ITEM:	SERVING:
		BREAKFAST	
○	60	EGG Substitute	1/2 Cup
○	150	Pork Chop (lean)	1
○	80	Fried Apples	1 Cup
○	20	Tomato Juice	4 oz.
○	60	Grapefruit	1/2
	370	**Breakfast Total**	
		Snack 1	
○	60	Cottage Cheese	4 TBSP
○	68	Strawberries	1 Cup
	128	**Snack 1 Total**	
		Lunch	
○	170	CHICKEN BRST (2)	7.5 oz.
○	40	Green SALAD	2 Cups
○	10	Mom's DRESSING	2 oz.
○	35	Apple Sliced	1/2 med
	255	**Lunch Total**	
		Snack 2	
○	50	Pudding (NS)	4 oz.
○	20	Blueberries	1/2 Cup
	70	**Snack 2 Total**	
		Dinner	
○	185	Round STEAK	3.75 oz.
○	30	Green SALAD	1.5 Cups
○	10	Mom's DRESSING	2 oz.
○	75	Apple	1 med
	300	**Dinner Total**	
		Snack 3	
○	50	Pudding (NS)	4 oz.
○	20	BlueBerries	1/2 Cup
	70	**Snack 3 Total**	

1193 TODAY'S Calorie TOTAL

DAY 5 — 1200

DATE:

Record YOUR MORNING Weight:

✓	C:	ITEM:	SERVING:
		BREAKFAST	
○	60	EGG Substitute	1/2 Cup
○	100	Chicken Sausage	1
○	70	Applesauce*	6 oz.
○	20	Tomato Juice	4 oz.
○	60	Grapefruit	1/2
	310	**Breakfast Total**	
		Snack 1	
○	100	Pudding (NS)	8 oz.
○	38	Peach slices (NS)	1 med
	138	**Snack 1 Total**	
		Lunch	
○	185	Round STEAK	3.75 oz.
○	40	Spinach SALAD	2 Cups
○	10	Mom's DRESSING	2 oz.
○	75	Apple Sliced	1 med
	294	**Lunch Total**	
		Snack 2	
○	60	Cottage Cheese	4 TBSP
○	18	Celery	1 Cup
	78	**Snack 2 Total**	
		Dinner	
○	170	CHICKEN BRST	7.5 oz.
○	40	Green SALAD/drsg	1.5 Cups
○	55	Blackberries	1 Cup
○	40	Blueberies	1 Cup
	280	**Dinner Total**	
		Snack 3	
○	50	Pudding (NS)	4 oz.
○	50	Raspberries	1 Cup
	100	**Snack 2 Total**	

1200 TODAY'S Calorie TOTAL

DAY 6 — 1200

DATE:

Record YOUR MORNING Weight:

✓	C:	ITEM:	SERVING:
		BREAKFAST	
○	185	Steak (lean)	3.75 oz.
○	20	Blueberries	1/2 Cup
○	70	Applesauce	6 oz.
○	50	V8 Juice	8 oz.
○	34	Strawberries	1/2 Cup
	359	**Breakfast Total**	
		Snack 1	
○	50	Raspberries	1 Cup
○	50	Pudding (NS)	4 oz.
	100	**Snack 1 Total**	
		Lunch	
○	170	CHICKEN BRST (2)	7.5 oz.
○	40	Green SALAD	2 Cups
○	10	Mom's DRESSING	2 oz.
○	68	Strawberries (NS)	1 Cup
	288	**Lunch Total**	
		Snack 2	
○	60	Cottage Cheese	4 TBSP
○	55	Blackberries (NS)	1 Cup
	115	**Snack 2 Total**	
		Dinner	
○	200	Chicken Sausages	2 oz.
○	30	Green SALAD	1.5 Cups
○	10	Mom's DRESSING	2 oz.
○	38	Peach Sliced	1 med
	278	**Dinner Total**	
		Snack 3	
○	50	Pudding (NS)	4 oz.
○	28	Blackberries	1/2 Cup
	70	**Snack 2 Total**	

1210 TODAY'S Calorie TOTAL

ISBN 978-0-9800641-8-6

'NO Sugar & Starch Diet Victory' EZPLAN™ | 1300 Calories

Day 1

DATE: _____

1300 **1**   Record YOUR MORNING Weight: _____

✓	C:	ITEM:	SERVING:
BREAKFAST			
○	60	EGG Substitute	1/2 Cup
○	102	BACON Slice	3
○	70	Applesauce*	6 oz.
○	50	V8 Juice	8 oz.
○	60	Grapefruit	1/2
	342	**Breakfast Total**	
Snack 1			
○	60	Cottage Cheese	4 TBSP
○	68	Strawberries	1 Cup
	128	**Snack 1 Total**	
Lunch			
○	170	CHICKEN BRST(2)	7.5 oz.
○	40	Green SALAD	2 Cups
○	10	Mom's DRESSING	2 oz.
○	40	Blueberries	1 Cup
	260	**Lunch Total**	
Snack 2			
○	100	Pudding (NS)	8 oz.
○			
	100	**Snack 2 Total**	
Dinner			
○	185	Round STEAK	3.75 oz.
○	40	Spinach SALAD	2 Cups
○	10	Mom's DRESSING	2 oz.
○	105	Apple Sauce (NS)	8 oz.
	340	**Dinner Total**	
Snack 3			
○	50	Pudding (NS)	7.5 oz.
○	76	Peach slices (NS)	2 med
	126	**Snack 3 Total**	

1296 TODAY'S Calorie TOTAL

Day 2

DATE: _____

1300 **2**   Record YOUR MORNING Weight: _____

✓	C:	ITEM:	SERVING:
BREAKFAST			
○	152	POACHED EGGS	2 Large
○	100	Chicken Sausage	1
○	35	Applesauce*	3 oz.
○	20	Tomato Juice	4 oz.
○	60	Grapefruit	1/2
	367	**Breakfast Total**	
Snack 1			
○	50	Pudding (NS)	4 oz.
○	40	BlueBerries	1 Cup
	90	**Snack 1 Total**	
Lunch			
○	180	FISH (lean)	8 oz.
○	40	Spinach SALAD	2 Cups
○	10	Mom's DRESSING	2 oz.
○	40	Blueberries	1 med
	270	**Lunch Total**	
Snack 2			
○	120	Cottage Cheese	8 TBSP
○	50	Raspberries	1 Cup
	170	**Snack 2 Total**	
Dinner			
○	170	CHICKEN BRST	7.5 oz.
○	30	Green SALAD	1.5 Cups
○	10	Mom's DRESSING	2 oz.
○	68	Strawberries	1 Cup
	278	**Dinner Total**	
Snack 3			
○	100	Pudding (NS)	8 oz.
○	28	Blackberries (NS)	1/2 Cup
	128	**Snack 2 Total**	

1303 TODAY'S Calorie TOTAL

Day 3

DATE: _____

1300 **3**   Record YOUR MORNING Weight: _____

✓	C:	ITEM:	SERVING:
BREAKFAST			
○	76	POACHED EGGS	1 Large
○	150	PORK Chop (lean)	3.75 oz
○	70	Applesauce	6 oz.
○	50	V8 Juice	8 oz.
○	40	BlueBerries	1 Cup
	386	**Breakfast Total**	
Snack 1			
○	50	Raspberries	1 Cup
○	50	Pudding (NS)	4 oz.
	100	**Snack 1 Total**	
Lunch			
○	170	CHICKEN BRST (2)	7.5 oz.
○	40	Green SALAD	2 Cups
○	10	Mom's DRESSING	2 oz.
○	68	Strawberries (NS)	1 Cup
	288	**Lunch Total**	
Snack 2			
○	120	Cottage Cheese	8 TBSP
○	76	Peach slices (NS)	2 Cups
	198	**Snack 2 Total**	
Dinner			
○	185	Round STEAK	3.75 oz.
○	30	Green SALAD	1.5 Cups
○	10	Mom's DRESSING	2 oz.
○	34	Strawberries	1/2 Cup
	259	**Dinner Total**	
Snack 3			
○	50	Pudding (NS)	1/2 Large
○	20	BlueBerries	1/2 Cup
	70	**Snack 2 Total**	

1301 TODAY'S Calorie TOTAL

'NO Sugar & Starch Diet Victory' EZPLAN™   1300 Calories

DAY 4 — 1300

DATE:

Record YOUR MORNING Weight:

✓	C:	ITEM:	SERVING:
BREAKFAST			
○	152	POACHED EGGS	2 Large
○	68	BACON Slice	2
○	70	Applesauce	6 oz.
○	50	V8 Juice	8 oz.
○	60	Grapefruit	1/2
	400	**Breakfast Total**	
Snack 1			
○	60	Cottage Cheese	4 TBSP
○	40	BlueBerries	1 Cup
	100	**Snack 1 Total**	
Lunch			
○	170	CHICKEN BRST(2)	7.5 oz.
○	40	Green SALAD	2 Cups
○	10	Mom's DRESSING	2 oz.
○	55	Blackberries	1 Cup
	275	**Lunch Total**	
Snack 2			
○	50	Pudding (NS)	4 oz.
○	68	Strawberries (NS)	1 Cup
	118	**Snack 2 Total**	
Dinner			
○	185	Round STEAK	3.75 oz.
○	30	Spinach SALAD	1.5 Cups
○	10	Mom's DRESSING	2 oz.
○	75	Apple Slices	1 med
	300	**Dinner Total**	
Snack 3			
○	100	Pudding (NS)	8 oz.
○	20	BlueBerries	1/2 Cup
	120	**Snack 3 Total**	

1313 TODAY'S Calorie TOTAL

DAY 5 — 1300

DATE:

Record YOUR MORNING Weight:

✓	C:	ITEM:	SERVING:
BREAKFAST			
○	152	POACHED EGGS	2 Large
○	100	Chicken Sausage	1
○	70	Applesauce	6 oz.
○	20	Tomato Juice	4 oz.
○	60	Grapefruit	1/2
	402	**Breakfast Total**	
Snack 1			
○	50	Pudding (NS)	4 oz.
○	68	Strawberries	1 Cup
	118	**Snack 1 Total**	
Lunch			
○	185	Round STEAK	3.75 oz.
○	40	Spinach SALAD	2 Cups
○	10	Mom's DRESSING	2 oz.
○	75	Apple Sliced	1 med
	294	**Lunch Total**	
Snack 2			
○	120	Cottage Cheese	8 TBSP
○	40	Blueberries	1 Cup
	160	**Snack 2 Total**	
Dinner			
○	180	FISH (lean)	8 oz.
○	30	Green SALAD	1.5 Cups
○	10	Mom's DRESSING	2 oz.
○	34	Strawberries	1/2 Cup
	254	**Dinner Total**	
Snack 3			
○	50	Pudding (NS)	7.5 oz.
○	28	Blackberries (NS)	1/2 Cup
	78	**Snack 2 Total**	

1306 TODAY'S Calorie TOTAL

DAY 6 — 1300

DATE:

Record YOUR MORNING Weight:

✓	C:	ITEM:	SERVING:
BREAKFAST			
○	120	EGG Substitute	1 Cup
○	40	BlueBerries	1 Cup
○	90	Applesauce	8 oz.
○	50	V8 Juice	8 oz.
○	68	Strawberries	1 Cup
	368	**Breakfast Total**	
Snack 1			
○	50	Raspberries	1 Cup
○	100	Pudding (NS)	8 oz.
	150	**Snack 1 Total**	
Lunch			
○	170	CHICKEN BRST (2)	7.5 oz.
○	40	Green SALAD	2 Cups
○	10	Mom's DRESSING	2 oz.
○	68	Strawberries (NS)	1 Cup
	288	**Lunch Total**	
Snack 2			
○	120	Cottage Cheese	8 TBSP
○	28	Blackberries (NS)	2 Cups
	148	**Snack 2 Total**	
Dinner			
○	185	Round STEAK	3.75 oz.
○	40	Green SALAD	2 Cups
○	10	Mom's DRESSING	2 oz.
○	38	Peach Slices	1 med
	273	**Dinner Total**	
Snack 3			
○	50	Pudding (NS)	1/2 Large
○	20	BlueBerries	1/2 Cup
	70	**Snack 2 Total**	

1297 TODAY'S Calorie TOTAL

'NO Sugar & Starch Diet Victory' EZPLAN™   1400 Calories

Day 1

DATE:

1400 · 1 — Record YOUR MORNING Weight:

✓	C:	ITEM:	SERVING:
		BREAKFAST	
○	120	EGG Substitute	1 Cup
○	102	BACON Slice	3
○	90	Applesauce	8 oz.
○	50	V8 Juice	8 oz.
○	60	Grapefruit	1/2
	422	**Breakfast Total**	
		Snack 1	
○	60	Cottage Cheese	4 TBSP
○	40	BlueBerries	1 Cup
	100	**Snack 1 Total**	
		Lunch	
○	170	CHICKEN BRST (2)	7.5 oz.
○	40	Green SALAD	2 Cups
○	10	Mom's DRESSING	2 oz.
○	75	Apple Sliced	1 med
	295	**Lunch Total**	
		Snack 2	
○	100	Pudding (NS)	8 oz.
○	68	Strawberries (NS)	1 Cup
	168	**Snack 2 Total**	
		Dinner	
○	185	Round STEAK	3.75 oz.
○	30	Spinach SALAD	1.5 Cups
○	10	Mom's DRESSING	2 oz.
○	90	Apple Sauce (NS)	8 oz.
	305	**Dinner Total**	
		Snack 3	
○	100	Pudding (NS)	7.5 oz.
○	20	BlueBerries	1/2 Cup
	120	**Snack 3 Total**	

1410 TODAY'S Calorie TOTAL

Day 2

DATE:

1400 · 2 — Record YOUR MORNING Weight:

✓	C:	ITEM:	SERVING:
		BREAKFAST	
○	152	POACHED EGGS	2 Large
○	200	Chicken Sausage	2
○	70	Applesauce	6 oz.
○	20	Tomato Juice	4 oz.
○	60	Grapefruit	1/2
	502	**Breakfast Total**	
		Snack 1	
○	50	Pudding (NS)	4 oz.
○	40	BlueBerries	1 Cup
	90	**Snack 1 Total**	
		Lunch	
○	185	Round STEAK	3.75 oz.
○	40	Spinach SALAD	2 Cups
○	10	Mom's DRESSING	2 oz.
○	75	Apple Sliced	1 med
	294	**Lunch Total**	
		Snack 2	
○	60	Cottage Cheese	4 TBSP
○	68	Strawberries (NS)	1 Cups
	128	**Snack 2 Total**	
		Dinner	
○	170	CHICKEN BRST	7.5 oz.
○	40	Green SALAD	2 Cups
○	10	Mom's DRESSING	2 oz.
○	70	Apple Fresh Sliced	1 med
	280	**Dinner Total**	
		Snack 3	
○	100	Pudding (NS)	8 oz.
○			
	100	**Snack 2 Total**	

1404 TODAY'S Calorie TOTAL

Day 3

DATE:

1400 · 3 — Record YOUR MORNING Weight:

✓	C:	ITEM:	SERVING:
		BREAKFAST	
○	152	POACHED EGGS	2 Large
○	40	BlueBerries	1 Cup
○	70	Applesauce*	6 oz.
○	50	V8 Juice	8 oz.
○	34	Strawberries	1/2 Cup
	346	**Breakfast Total**	
		Snack 1	
○	50	Raspberries	1 Cup
○	100	Pudding (NS)	8 oz.
	150	**Snack 1 Total**	
		Lunch	
○	170	CHICKEN BRST (2)	7.5 oz.
○	40	Green SALAD	2 Cups
○	10	Mom's DRESSING	2 oz.
○	68	Strawberries (NS)	1 Cup
	288	**Lunch Total**	
		Snack 2	
○	120	Cottage Cheese	8 TBSP
○	55	Blackberries (NS)	2 Cups
	175	**Snack 2 Total**	
		Dinner	
○	185	Round STEAK	3.75 oz.
○	30	Green SALAD	1.5 Cups
○	10	Mom's DRESSING	2 oz.
○	76	Peaches Sliced	2 med
	301	**Dinner Total**	
		Snack 3	
○	100	Pudding (NS)	8 oz.
○	40	BlueBerries	1 Cup
	140	**Snack 2 Total**	

1400 TODAY'S Calorie TOTAL

'NO Sugar & Starch Diet Victory' EZPLAN™ | 1400 Calories

DATE: **DATE:**   **DATE:**

Day 4 (1400) — Record YOUR MORNING Weight:

✓	C:	ITEM:	SERVING:
		BREAKFAST	
○	120	EGG Substitue	1 Cup
○	102	BACON Slice	3
○	70	Applesauce	6 oz.
○	50	V8 Juice	8 oz.
○	60	Grapefruit	1/2
	402	Breakfast Total	
		Snack 1	
○	120	Cottage Cheese	8 TBSP
○	40	BlueBerries	1 Cup
	160	Snack 1 Total	
		Lunch	
○	170	CHICKEN BRST(2)	7.5 oz.
○	40	Green SALAD	2 Cups
○	10	Mom's DRESSING	2 oz.
○	75	Apple Sliced	1 med
	295	Lunch Total	
		Snack 2	
○	100	Pudding (NS)	8 oz.
○	68	Strawberries (NS)	1 Cup
	168	Snack 2 Total	
		Dinner	
○	185	Round STEAK	3.75 oz.
○	30	Spinach SALAD	1.5 Cups
○	10	Mom's DRESSING	2 oz.
○	70	Apple Sauce (NS)	6 oz.
	295	Dinner Total	
		Snack 3	
○	50	Pudding (NS)	4 oz.
○	40	BlueBerries	1 Cup
	90	Snack 3 Total	

1410   TODAY'S Calorie TOTAL

Day 5 (1400) — Record YOUR MORNING Weight:

✓	C:	ITEM:	SERVING:
		BREAKFAST	
○	76	POACHED EGG	1 Large
○	200	Chicken Sausage	2
○	90	Applesauce	8 oz.
○	20	Tomato Juice	4 oz.
○	60	Grapefruit	1/2
	446	Breakfast Total	
		Snack 1	
○	50	Pudding (NS)	4 oz.
○	40	BlueBerries	1 Cup
	90	Snack 1 Total	
		Lunch	
○	185	Round STEAK	3.75 oz.
○	40	Spinach SALAD	2 Cups
○	10	Mom's DRESSING	2 oz.
○	75	Apple Sliced	1 med
	294	Lunch Total	
		Snack 2	
○	120	Cottage Cheese	8 TBSP
○	68	Strawberries (NS)	1 Cups
	188	Snack 2 Total	
		Dinner	
○	170	CHICKEN BRST	7.5 oz.
○	30	Green SALAD	1.5 Cups
○	10	Mom's DRESSING	2 oz.
○	70	Apple Fresh Sliced	1 med
	280	Dinner Total	
		Snack 3	
○	50	Pudding (NS)	7.5 oz.
○	56	Blackberries (NS)	1 Cup
	106	Snack 2 Total	

1404   TODAY'S Calorie TOTAL

Day 6 (1400) — Record YOUR MORNING Weight:

✓	C:	ITEM:	SERVING:
		BREAKFAST	
○	150	PORK Chop	3 oz.
○	40	BlueBerries	1 Cup
○	70	Applesauce	6 oz.
○	50	V8 Juice	8 oz.
○	68	Strawberries	1 Cup
	378	Breakfast Total	
		Snack 1	
○	50	Raspberries	1 Cup
○	100	Pudding (NS)	8 oz.
	150	Snack 1 Total	
		Lunch	
○	170	CHICKEN BRST (2)	7.5 oz.
○	40	Green SALAD	2 Cups
○	10	Mom's DRESSING	2 oz.
○	68	Strawberries (NS)	1 Cup
	288	Lunch Total	
		Snack 2	
○	120	Cottage Cheese	8 TBSP
○	55	Blackberries (NS)	2 Cups
	175	Snack 2 Total	
		Dinner	
○	185	Round STEAK	3.75 oz.
○	30	Green SALAD	1.5 Cups
○	10	Mom's DRESSING	2 oz.
○	38	Peach Sliced	1 med
	263	Dinner Total	
		Snack 3	
○	100	Pudding (NS)	8 oz.
○	40	BlueBerries	1 Cup
	140	Snack 2 Total	

1394   TODAY'S Calorie TOTAL

'NO Sugar & Starch Diet Victory' EZPLAN™ | 1500 Calories

Day 1

DATE:

1500 **1** — Record YOUR MORNING Weight:

✓	C:	ITEM:	SERVING:
BREAKFAST			
○	152	POACHED EGGS	2 Large
○	136	BACON Slice	4
○	70	Applesauce*	6 oz.
○	50	V8 Juice	8 oz.
○	60	Grapefruit	1/2
	468	**Breakfast Total**	
Snack 1			
○	120	Cottage Cheese	8 TBSP
○	40	BlueBerries	1 Cup
	160	**Snack 1 Total**	
Lunch			
○	170	CHICKEN BRST (2)	7.5 oz.
○	40	Green SALAD	2 Cups
○	10	Mom's DRESSING	2 oz.
○	75	Apple Sliced	1 med
	295	**Lunch Total**	
Snack 2			
○	100	Pudding (NS)	8 oz.
○	68	Strawberries (NS)	1 Cup
	168	**Snack 2 Total**	
Dinner			
○	185	Round STEAK	3.75 oz.
○	30	Spinach SALAD	1.5 Cups
○	10	Mom's DRESSING	2 oz.
○	100	Apple Sauce (NS)	8 oz.
	325	**Dinner Total**	
Snack 3			
○	50	Pudding (NS)	4 oz.
○	40	BlueBerries	1 Cup
	90	**Snack 3 Total**	

1506   TODAY'S Calorie TOTAL

Day 2

DATE:

1500 **2** — Record YOUR MORNING Weight:

✓	C:	ITEM:	SERVING:
BREAKFAST			
○	120	EGG Substitute	1 Cup
○	200	Chicken Sausage	2
○	100	Fried Apples (NS)	6 oz.
○	40	Tomato Juice	8 oz.
○			1/2
	460	**Breakfast Total**	
Snack 1			
○	100	Pudding (NS)	8 oz.
○	40	BlueBerries	1 Cup
	140	**Snack 1 Total**	
Lunch			
○	185	Round STEAK	3.75 oz.
○	40	Spinach SALAD	2 Cups
○	10	Mom's DRESSING	2 oz.
○	150	Apple Sliced	2 med
	385	**Lunch Total**	
Snack 2			
○	60	Cottage Cheese	4 TBSP
○	68	Strawberries (NS)	1 Cups
	128	**Snack 2 Total**	
Dinner			
○	170	CHICKEN BRST	7.5 oz.
○	40	Green SALAD	2 Cups
○	10	Mom's DRESSING	2 oz.
○	70	Apple Fresh Sliced	1 med
	290	**Dinner Total**	
Snack 3			
○	50	Pudding (NS)	7.5 oz.
○	55	Blackberries (NS)	1 Cup
	105	**Snack 2 Total**	

1508   TODAY'S Calorie TOTAL

Day 3

DATE:

1500 **3** — Record YOUR MORNING Weight:

✓	C:	ITEM:	SERVING:
BREAKFAST			
○	152	POACHED EGGS	2 Large
○	40	BlueBerries	1 Cup
○	100	Applesauce	80 oz.
○	50	V8 Juice	8 oz.
○	68	Strawberries	1 Cup
	410	**Breakfast Total**	
Snack 1			
○	50	Raspberries	1 Cup
○	100	Pudding (NS)	8 oz.
	150	**Snack 1 Total**	
Lunch			
○	170	CHICKEN BRST (2)	7.5 oz.
○	40	Green SALAD	2 Cups
○	10	Mom's DRESSING	2 oz.
○	102	Strawberries (NS)	1 1/2 Cups
	322	**Lunch Total**	
Snack 2			
○	120	Cottage Cheese	8 TBSP
○	55	Blackberries (NS)	2 Cups
	175	**Snack 2 Total**	
Dinner			
○	185	Round STEAK	3.75 oz.
○	40	Green SALAD	2 Cups
○	10	Mom's DRESSING	2 oz.
○	76	Peaches Sliced	2 med
	311	**Dinner Total**	
Snack 3			
○	100	Pudding (NS)	1/2 Large
○	40	BlueBerries	1/2 Cup
	140	**Snack 2 Total**	

1508   TODAY'S Calorie TOTAL

'NO Sugar & Starch Diet Victory' EZPLAN™ — 1500 Calories

DAY 4 — 1500

Record YOUR MORNING Weight:

C:	ITEM:	SERVING:
BREAKFAST		
120	EGG Substitiute	1 Cup
150	PORK Chop	3 oz.
100	Applesauce	8 oz.
50	V8 Juice	8 oz.
60	Grapefruit	1/2
480	**Breakfast Total**	
Snack 1		
60	Cottage Cheese	4 TBSP
40	BlueBerries	1 Cup
100	**Snack 1 Total**	
Lunch		
170	CHICKEN BRST(2)	7.5 oz.
40	Green SALAD	2 Cups
10	Mom's DRESSING	2 oz.
75	Apple Sliced	1 med
295	**Lunch Total**	
Snack 2		
100	Pudding (NS)	8 oz.
68	Strawberries (NS)	1 Cup
168	**Snack 2 Total**	
Dinner		
185	Round STEAK	3.75 oz.
30	Spinach SALAD	1.5 Cups
10	Mom's DRESSING	2 oz.
100	Apple Sauce (NS)	8 oz.
325	**Dinner Total**	
Snack 3		
100	Pudding (NS)	8 oz.
40	BlueBerries	1 Cup
140	**Snack 3 Total**	

1508 TODAY'S Calorie TOTAL

DAY 5 — 1500

Record YOUR MORNING Weight:

C:	ITEM:	SERVING:
BREAKFAST		
152	POACHED EGGS	2 Large
100	Chicken Sausage	1
100	Applesauce	8 oz.
40	Tomato Juice	8 oz.
60	Grapefruit	1/2
452	**Breakfast Total**	
Snack 1		
100	Pudding (NS)	8 oz.
40	BlueBerries	1 Cup
140	**Snack 1 Total**	
Lunch		
185	Round STEAK	3.75 oz.
40	Spinach SALAD	2 Cups
10	Mom's DRESSING	2 oz.
75	Apple Sliced	1 med
294	**Lunch Total**	
Snack 2		
100	Chicken Sausage	1
70	Applesauce	6 oz.
170	**Snack 2 Total**	
Dinner		
170	CHICKEN BRST	7.5 oz.
40	Green SALAD	2 Cups
10	Mom's DRESSING	2 oz.
70	Apple Fresh Sliced	1 med
290	**Dinner Total**	
Snack 3		
100	Pudding (NS)	8 oz.
55	Blackberries (NS)	1 Cup
155	**Snack 2 Total**	

1501 TODAY'S Calorie TOTAL

DAY 6 — 1500

Record YOUR MORNING Weight:

C:	ITEM:	SERVING:
BREAKFAST		
228	POACHED EGGS	3 Large
40	BlueBerries	1 Cup
70	Applesauce	6 oz.
50	V8 Juice	8 oz.
68	Strawberries	1 Cup
456	**Breakfast Total**	
Snack 1		
50	Raspberries	1 Cup
100	Pudding (NS)	8 oz.
150	**Snack 1 Total**	
Lunch		
170	CHICKEN BRST (2)	7.5 oz.
40	Green SALAD	2 Cups
10	Mom's DRESSING	2 oz.
68	Strawberries (NS)	1 Cup
288	**Lunch Total**	
Snack 2		
120	Cottage Cheese	8 TBSP
55	Blackberries (NS)	1 Cups
175	**Snack 2 Total**	
Dinner		
185	Round STEAK	3.75 oz.
40	Green SALAD	2 Cups
10	Mom's DRESSING	2 oz.
38	Peach Sliced	1 med
273	**Dinner Total**	
Snack 3		
100	Pudding (NS)	1/2 Large
55	BlueBerries	1/2 Cup
155	**Snack 2 Total**	

1497 TODAY'S Calorie TOTAL

'NO Sugar & Starch Diet Victory' EZPLAN™   1600 Calories

Day 1

DATE:

1600 **1**

Record YOUR MORNING Weight:

✓	C:	ITEM:	SERVING:
		BREAKFAST	
○	152	POACHED EGGS	2 Large
○	102	BACON Slice	3
○	70	Applesauce	6 oz.
○	50	V8 Juice	8 oz.
○	60	Grapefruit	1/2
	434	**Breakfast Total**	
		Snack 1	
○	120	Cottage Cheese	8 TBSP
○	40	BlueBerries	1 Cup
	160	**Snack 1 Total**	
		Lunch	
○	170	CHICKEN BRST(2)	7.5 oz.
○	40	Green SALAD	2 Cups
○	10	Mom's DRESSING	2 oz.
○	68	Strawberries	1 Cup
	288	**Lunch Total**	
		Snack 2	
○	50	Pudding (NS)	4 oz.
○	55	Blackberries	1 Cup
	105	**Snack 2 Total**	
		Dinner	
○	370	Round STEAKS (2)	7.5 oz.
○	30	Spinach SALAD	1.5 Cups
○	10	Mom's DRESSING	2 oz.
○	70	Apple Sauce (NS)	6 oz.
	480	**Dinner Total**	
		Snack 3	
○	100	Pudding (NS)	8 oz.
○	40	BlueBerries	1 Cup
	140	**Snack 3 Total**	

1607   TODAY'S Calorie TOTAL

Day 2

DATE:

1600 **2**

Record YOUR MORNING Weight:

✓	C:	ITEM:	SERVING:
		BREAKFAST	
○	152	POACHED EGGS	2 Large
○	100	Chicken Sausage	1
○	100	Applesauce	8 oz.
○	40	Tomato Juice	8 oz.
○	60	Grapefruit	1/2
	452	**Breakfast Total**	
		Snack 1	
○	100	Pudding (NS)	4 oz.
○	40	BlueBerries	1 Cup
	140	**Snack 1 Total**	
		Lunch	
○	185	Round STEAK	3.75 oz.
○	40	Spinach SALAD	2 Cups
○	10	Mom's DRESSING	2 oz.
○	150	Apple Slices	2 med
	385	**Lunch Total**	
		Snack 2	
○	120	Cottage Cheese	8 TBSP
○	68	Strawberries (NS)	1 Cups
	188	**Snack 2 Total**	
		Dinner	
○	270	FISH low fat (3)	11.25 oz.
○	30	Green SALAD	1.5 Cups
○	10	Mom's DRESSING	2 oz.
○	20	Blueberries	1/2 Cup
	330	**Dinner Total**	
		Snack 3	
○	50	Pudding (NS)	7.5 oz.
○	55	Blackberries (NS)	1/2 Cup
	105	**Snack 2 Total**	

1600   TODAY'S Calorie TOTAL

Day 3

DATE:

1600 **3**

Record YOUR MORNING Weight:

✓	C:	ITEM:	SERVING:
		BREAKFAST	
○	120	EGG Substitute	1 Cup
○	150	PORK Chop	3 oz.
○	100	Applesauce	8 oz.
○	50	V8 Juice	8 oz.
○	68	Strawberries	1 Cup
	488	**Breakfast Total**	
		Snack 1	
○	50	Raspberries	1 Cup
○	100	Pudding (NS)	8 oz.
	150	**Snack 1 Total**	
		Lunch	
○	255	CHICKEN BRST (3)	11.25 oz.
○	40	Green SALAD	2 Cups
○	10	Mom's DRESSING	2 oz.
○	68	Strawberries (NS)	1 Cup
	373	**Lunch Total**	
		Snack 2	
○	120	Cottage Cheese	8 TBSP
○	55	Blackberries (NS)	1 Cup
	175	**Snack 2 Total**	
		Dinner	
○	185	Round STEAK	3.75 oz.
○	30	Green SALAD	1.5 Cups
○	10	Mom's DRESSING	2 oz.
○	76	Peaches Sliced	2 med
	301	**Dinner Total**	
		Snack 3	
○	100	Pudding (NS)	8 oz.
○	20	BlueBerries	1/2 Cup
	120	**Snack 2 Total**	

1607   TODAY'S Calorie TOTAL

'NO Sugar & Starch Diet Victory' EZPLAN™   1600 Calories

DAY 4

DATE:

1600 / 4

Record YOUR MORNING Weight:

✓	C:	ITEM:	SERVING:
BREAKFAST			
○	152	POACHED EGGS	2 Large
○	136	BACON Slice	4
○	100	Applesauce	8 oz.
○	50	V8 Juice	8 oz.
○	60	Grapefruit	1/2
	498	**Breakfast Total**	
Snack 1			
○	120	Cottage Cheese	8 TBSP
○	40	BlueBerries	1 Cup
	160	**Snack 1 Total**	
Lunch			
○	170	CHICKEN BRST (2)	7.5 oz.
○	40	Green SALAD	2 Cups
○	10	Mom's DRESSING	2 oz.
○	143	Apple & Berries	1 med
	363	**Lunch Total**	
Snack 2			
○	100	Pudding (NS)	4 oz.
○	34	Strawberries (NS)	1/2 Cup
	134	**Snack 2 Total**	
Dinner			
○	185	Round STEAK	3.75 oz.
○	30	Spinach SALAD	1.5 Cups
○	10	Mom's DRESSING	2 oz.
○	100	Apple Sauce (NS)	8 oz.
	325	**Dinner Total**	
Snack 3			
○	100	Pudding (NS)	7.5 oz.
○	20	BlueBerries	1/2 Cup
	120	**Snack 3 Total**	

1600   TODAY'S Calorie TOTAL

DAY 5

DATE:

1600 / 5

Record YOUR MORNING Weight:

✓	C:	ITEM:	SERVING:
BREAKFAST			
○	152	POACHED EGGS	2 Large
○	150	PORK Chop	3 oz.
○	100	Applesauce	8 oz.
○	20	Tomato Juice	4 oz.
○	60	Grapefruit	1/2
	482	**Breakfast Total**	
Snack 1			
○	100	Pudding (NS)	8 oz.
○	40	BlueBerries	1 Cup
	140	**Snack 1 Total**	
Lunch			
○	370	Round STEAK (2)	7.5 oz.
○	40	Spinach SALAD	2 Cups
○	10	Mom's DRESSING	2 oz.
○	75	Apple Sliced	1 med
	495	**Lunch Total**	
Snack 2			
○	60	Cottage Cheese	4 TBSP
○	68	Strawberries (NS)	1/2 Cup
	128	**Snack 2 Total**	
Dinner			
○	170	CHICKEN BRST	7.5 oz.
○	30	Green SALAD	1.5 Cups
○	10	Mom's DRESSING	2 oz.
○	40	BlueBerries	1 Cup
	250	**Dinner Total**	
Snack 3			
○	50	Pudding (NS)	4 oz.
○	55	Blackberries (NS)	1/2 Cup
	105	**Snack 2 Total**	

1600   TODAY'S Calorie TOTAL

DAY 6

DATE:

1600 / 6

Record YOUR MORNING Weight:

✓	C:	ITEM:	SERVING:
BREAKFAST			
○	152	POACHED EGGS	2 Large
○	185	Steak	3.75 oz.
○	70	Applesauce	6 oz.
○	50	V8 Juice	8 oz.
○	34	Strawberries	1/2 Cup
	491	**Breakfast Total**	
Snack 1			
○	50	Raspberries	1 Cup
○	100	Pudding (NS)	8 oz.
	150	**Snack 1 Total**	
Lunch			
○	170	CHICKEN BRST (2)	7.5 oz.
○	40	Green SALAD	2 Cups
○	10	Mom's DRESSING	2 oz.
○	143	Apple & Berries	1 Cup
	363	**Lunch Total**	
Snack 2			
○	120	Cottage Cheese	8 TBSP
○	55	Blackberries (NS)	2 Cups
	175	**Snack 2 Total**	
Dinner			
○	270	FISH Lean (3)	11.25 oz.
○	30	Green SALAD	1.5 Cups
○	10	Mom's DRESSING	2 oz.
○	38	Peach Sliced	1 med
	348	**Dinner Total**	
Snack 3			
○	50	Pudding (NS)	1/2 Large
○	20	BlueBerries	1/2 Cup
	70	**Snack 2 Total**	

1597   TODAY'S Calorie TOTAL

'NO Sugar & Starch Diet Victory' EZPLAN™   1700 Calories

DAY 1 — 1700

DATE:

Record YOUR MORNING Weight:

✓	C:	ITEM:	SERVING:
		BREAKFAST	
○	152	POACHED EGGS	2 Large
○	136	BACON Slices	4
○	100	Applesauce	8 oz.
○	50	V8 Juice	8 oz.
○	60	Grapefruit	1/2
	498	**Breakfast Total**	
		Snack 1	
○	120	Cottage Cheese	8 TBSP
○	40	BlueBerries	1 Cup
	160	**Snack 1 Total**	
		Lunch	
○	170	CHICKEN BRST (2)	7.5 oz.
○	50	Grn SALAD & Drsg	2 Cups
○	28	Cherry TOMATOES	1 Cup
○	150	Apple Sliced	2 med
	398	**Lunch Total**	
		Snack 2	
○	100	Pudding (NS)	8 oz.
○	68	Strawberries (NS)	1 Cup
	168	**Snack 2 Total**	
		Dinner	
○	185	Round STEAK	3.75 oz.
○	40	Spinach SALAD	2 Cups
○	10	Mom's DRESSING	2 oz.
○	100	Apple Sauce (NS)	8 oz.
	335	**Dinner Total**	
		Snack 3	
○	100	Pudding (NS)	8 oz.
○	40	BlueBerries	1 Cup
	140	**Snack 3 Total**	

1699 TODAY'S Calorie TOTAL

DAY 2 — 1700

DATE:

Record YOUR MORNING Weight:

✓	C:	ITEM:	SERVING:
		BREAKFAST	
○	152	POACHED EGGS	2 Large
○	200	Chicken Sausages	2
○	100	Applesauce*	8 oz.
○	40	Tomato Juice	8 oz.
○	60	Grapefruit	1/2
	492	**Breakfast Total**	
		Snack 1	
○	100	Pudding (NS)	8 oz.
○	40	BlueBerries	1 Cup
	140	**Snack 1 Total**	
		Lunch	
○	370	Round STEAK (2)	7.5 oz.
○	40	Spinach SALAD	2 Cups
○	10	Mom's DRESSING	2 oz.
○	75	Apple Sliced	1 med
	495	**Lunch Total**	
		Snack 2	
○	120	Cottage Cheese	8 TBSP
○	68	Strawberries (NS)	1 Cups
	188	**Snack 2 Total**	
		Dinner	
○	170	CHICKEN BRST (2)	7.5 oz.
○	40	Grn. SALAD & Drsg	1.5 Cups
○	28	Mom's DRESSING	1 Cup
○	70	Apple Fresh Sliced	1 med
	308	**Dinner Total**	
		Snack 3	
○	50	Pudding (NS)	4 oz.
○	28	Blackberries (NS)	1/2 Cup
	78	**Snack 2 Total**	

1701 TODAY'S Calorie TOTAL

DAY 3 — 1700

DATE:

Record YOUR MORNING Weight:

✓	C:	ITEM:	SERVING:
		BREAKFAST	
○	120	EGG Substitute	1 Cup
○	40	BlueBerries	1 Cup
○	100	Applesauce*	8 oz.
○	50	V8 Juice	8 oz.
○	68	Strawberries	1 Cup
	378	**Breakfast Total**	
		Snack 1	
○	50	Raspberries	1 Cup
○	100	Pudding (NS)	8 oz.
	150	**Snack 1 Total**	
		Lunch	
○	255	CHICKEN BRST (3)	7.5 oz.
○	50	Grn. SALAD & Drsg	2 Cups
○	28	Cherry Tomatoes	1 Cup
○	55	Blackberries (NS)	1 Cup
	388	**Lunch Total**	
		Snack 2	
○	120	Cottage Cheese	8 TBSP
○	68	Strawberries (NS)	1 Cup
	188	**Snack 2 Total**	
		Dinner	
○	370	Round STEAK (2)	7.5 oz.
○	40	Grn. SALAD & Drsg	1.5 Cups
○	38	Green Beans	2 oz.
○	76	Peach Slices	2 med
	524	**Dinner Total**	
		Snack 3	
○	50	Pudding (NS)	1/2 Large
○	20	BlueBerries	1/2 Cup
	70	**Snack 2 Total**	

1698 TODAY'S Calorie TOTAL

'NO Sugar & Starch Diet Victory' EZPLAN™   1700 Calories

DAY 4 — 1700

DATE:

Record YOUR MORNING Weight:

✓	C:	ITEM:	SERVING:
BREAKFAST			
○	152	POACHED EGGs	2 Large
○	200	Chicken Sausages	2
○	70	Applesauce*	6 oz.
○	50	V8 Juice	8 oz.
○	60	Grapefruit	1/2
	532	Breakfast Total	
Snack 1			
○	120	Cottage Cheese	8 TBSP
○	40	BlueBerries	1 Cup
	160	Snack 1 Total	
Lunch			
○	170	CHICKEN BRST (2)	7.5 oz.
○	50	Green SALAD/Drsg	2 Cups
○	150	Apple Slices	2 med
○			
	370	Lunch Total	
Snack 2			
○	100	Pudding (NS)	8 oz.
○	68	Strawberries (NS)	1 Cup
	168	Snack 2 Total	
Dinner			
○	185	Round STEAK	3.75 oz.
○	30	Spinach SALAD	1.5 Cups
○	10	Mom's DRESSING	2 oz.
○	100	Apple Sauce (NS)	8 oz.
	325	Dinner Total	
Snack 3			
○	100	Pudding (NS)	8 oz.
○	40	BlueBerries	1 Cup
	140	Snack 3 Total	

1695   TODAY'S Calorie TOTAL

DAY 5 — 1700

DATE:

Record YOUR MORNING Weight:

✓	C:	ITEM:	SERVING:
BREAKFAST			
○	152	POACHED EGGS	2 Large
○	150	Lean Pork Chop	1
○	100	Applesauce*	8 oz.
○	40	Tomato Juice	8 oz.
○	60	Grapefruit	1/2
	502	Breakfast Total	
Snack 1			
○	100	Pudding (NS)	4 oz.
○	60	BlueBerries	1 1/2 Cups
	160	Snack 1 Total	
Lunch			
○	370	Round STEAK (2)	3.75 oz.
○	40	Spinach SALAD	2 Cups
○	10	Mom's DRESSING	2 oz.
○	75	Apple Sliced	1 med
	495	Lunch Total	
Snack 2			
○	120	Cottage Cheese	4 TBSP
○	68	Strawberries (NS)	1 Cups
	188	Snack 2 Total	
Dinner			
○	170	CHICKEN BRST (2)	7.5 oz.
○	30	Green SALAD	1.5 Cups
○	10	Mom's DRESSING	2 oz.
○	70	Apple Fresh Sliced	1 med
	280	Dinner Total	
Snack 3			
○	50	Pudding (NS)	7.5 oz.
○	28	Blackberries (NS)	1/2 Cup
	78	Snack 2 Total	

1703   TODAY'S Calorie TOTAL

DAY 6 — 1700

DATE:

Record YOUR MORNING Weight:

✓	C:	ITEM:	SERVING:
BREAKFAST			
○	152	POACHED EGGS	2 Large
○	185	Round STEAK	3.75 oz.
○	100	Applesauce*	8 oz.
○	50	V8 Juice	8 oz.
○	68	Strawberries	1 Cup
	555	Breakfast Total	
Snack 1			
○	50	Raspberries	1 Cup
○	100	Pudding (NS)	1 Cup
	150	Snack 1 Total	
Lunch			
○	170	CHICKEN BRST (2)	7.5 oz.
○	40	Green SALAD	2 Cups
○	10	Mom's DRESSING	2 oz.
○	68	Strawberries (NS)	1 Cup
	288	Lunch Total	
Snack 2			
○	120	Cottage Cheese	8 TBSP
○	55	Blackberries (NS)	2 Cups
	175	Snack 2 Total	
Dinner			
○	370	Round STEAK (2)	7.5 oz.
○	30	Green SALAD	1.5 Cups
○	10	Mom's DRESSING	2 oz.
○	38	Peach Sliced	1 med
	448	Dinner Total	
Snack 3			
○	50	Pudding (NS)	1/2 Large
○	40	BlueBerries	1 Cup
	90	Snack 2 Total	

1706   TODAY'S Calorie TOTAL

'NO Sugar & Starch Diet Victory' EZPLAN™ | 1800 Calories

Day 1 (1800)

DATE: _____

Record YOUR MORNING Weight: _____

✓	C:	ITEM:	SERVING:
		BREAKFAST	
○	152	POACHED EGGS	2 Large
○	150	Lean Pork Chop	3 oz.
○	100	Applesauce	8 oz.
○	50	V8 Juice	8 oz.
○	60	Grapefruit	1/2
	512	**Breakfast Total**	
		Snack 1	
○	120	Cottage Cheese	8 TBSP
○	40	BlueBerries	1 Cup
	160	**Snack 1 Total**	
		Lunch	
○	170	CHICKEN BRST (2)	7.5 oz.
○	40	Green SALAD	2 Cups
○	10	Mom's DRESSING	2 oz.
○	150	Apples Sliced	2 med
	370	**Lunch Total**	
		Snack 2	
○	100	Pudding (NS)	8 oz.
○	68	Strawberries (NS)	1 Cup
	168	**Snack 2 Total**	
		Dinner	
○	370	Round STEAK (2)	7.5 oz.
○	30	Spinach SALAD	1.5 Cups
○	10	Mom's DRESSING	2 oz.
○	100	Apple Sauce (NS)	6 oz.
	510	**Dinner Total**	
		Snack 3	
○	50	Pudding (NS)	7.5 oz.
○	40	BlueBerries	1 Cup
	90	**Snack 3 Total**	

1810 TODAY'S Calorie TOTAL

Day 2 (1800)

DATE: _____

Record YOUR MORNING Weight: _____

✓	C:	ITEM:	SERVING:
		BREAKFAST	
○	120	EGG Substitute	1 Cup
○	200	Chicken Sausage	2
○	100	Applesauce	6 oz.
○	40	Tomato Juice	4 oz.
○	60	Grapefruit	1/2
	552	**Breakfast Total**	
		Snack 1	
○	100	Pudding (NS)	4 oz.
○	40	BlueBerries	1 Cup
	140	**Snack 1 Total**	
		Lunch	
○	370	Round STEAK (2)	7.5 oz.
○	40	Spinach SALAD	2 Cups
○	10	Mom's DRESSING	2 oz.
○	75	Apple Sliced	1 med
	495	**Lunch Total**	
		Snack 2	
○	60	Cottage Cheese	4 TBSP
○	68	Strawberries (NS)	1 Cups
	128	**Snack 2 Total**	
		Dinner	
○	170	CHICKEN BRST	7.5 oz.
○	40	Green SALAD	2 Cups
○	10	Mom's DRESSING	2 oz.
○	140	Apples Sliced	2 med
	360	**Dinner Total**	
		Snack 3	
○	100	Pudding (NS)	8 oz.
○	28	Blackberries (NS)	1/2 Cup
	128	**Snack 2 Total**	

1803 TODAY'S Calorie TOTAL

Day 3 (1800)

DATE: _____

Record YOUR MORNING Weight: _____

✓	C:	ITEM:	SERVING:
		BREAKFAST	
○	152	POACHED EGGS	2 Large
○	150	Lean Pork Chop	3 oz.
○	100	Applesauce*	8 oz.
○	50	V8 Juice	8 oz.
○	68	Strawberries	1 Cup
	520	**Breakfast Total**	
		Snack 1	
○	50	Raspberries	1 Cup
○	100	Pudding (NS)	4 oz.
	150	**Snack 1 Total**	
		Lunch	
○	170	CHICKEN BRST (2)	7.5 oz.
○	40	Green SALAD	2 Cups
○	10	Mom's DRESSING	2 oz.
○	108	BBerries/StrawB	2 Cups
	328	**Lunch Total**	
		Snack 2	
○	120	Cottage Cheese	8 TBSP
○	55	Blackberries (NS)	1 Cup
	175	**Snack 2 Total**	
		Dinner	
○	370	Round STEAK (2)	7.5 oz.
○	30	Green SALAD	1.5 Cups
○	10	Mom's DRESSING	2 oz.
○	76	Peaches Sliced	2 med
	486	**Dinner Total**	
		Snack 3	
○	100	Pudding (NS)	8 oz
○	40	BlueBerries	1/2 Cup
	140	**Snack 2 Total**	

1799 TODAY'S Calorie TOTAL

'NO Sugar & Starch Diet Victory' EZPLAN™   1800 Calories

DAY 4

DATE:

1800 / 4

Record YOUR MORNING Weight:

C:	ITEM:	SERVING:
BREAKFAST		
152	POACHED EGGS	2 Large
200	Chicken Sausages	2
100	Applesauce	8 oz.
50	V8 Juice	8 oz.
60	Grapefruit	1/2
562	**Breakfast Total**	
Snack 1		
60	Cottage Cheese	4 TBSP
40	BlueBerries	1 Cup
100	**Snack 1 Total**	
Lunch		
170	CHICKEN BRST (2)	7.5 oz.
40	Green SALAD	2 Cups
10	Mom's DRESSING	2 oz.
150	Apples Sliced	2 med
370	**Lunch Total**	
Snack 2		
50	Pudding (NS)	4 oz.
68	Strawberries (NS)	1 Cup
118	**Snack 2 Total**	
Dinner		
370	Round STEAK	7.5 oz.
30	Spinach SALAD	1.5 Cups
10	Mom's DRESSING	2 oz.
100	Apple Sauce (NS)	8 oz.
510	**Dinner Total**	
Snack 3		
100	Pudding (NS)	8 oz.
40	BlueBerries	1 Cup
140	**Snack 3 Total**	

1800 TODAY'S Calorie TOTAL

DAY 5

DATE:

1800 / 5

Record YOUR MORNING Weight:

C:	ITEM:	SERVING:
BREAKFAST		
152	POACHED EGGS	2 Large
200	Chicken Sausages	2
100	Applesauce*	6 oz.
40	Tomato Juice	4 oz.
60	Grapefruit	1/2
552	**Breakfast Total**	
Snack 1		
100	Pudding (NS)	4 oz.
40	BlueBerries	1 Cup
140	**Snack 1 Total**	
Lunch		
370	Round STEAK	7.5 oz.
40	Spinach SALAD	2 Cups
10	Mom's DRESSING	2 oz.
75	Apple Sliced	1 med
495	**Lunch Total**	
Snack 2		
120	Cottage Cheese	4 TBSP
34	Strawberries (NS)	1/2 Cup
154	**Snack 2 Total**	
Dinner		
170	CHICKEN BRST (2)	7.5 oz.
40	Green SALAD/Drsg	1.5 Cups
40	Blueberries	1 Cup
140	Apples Sliced	2 med
390	**Dinner Total**	
Snack 3		
50	Pudding (NS)	7.5 oz.
28	Blackberries (NS)	1/2 Cup
78	**Snack 2 Total**	

1809 TODAY'S Calorie TOTAL

DAY 6

DATE:

1800 / 6

Record YOUR MORNING Weight:

C:	ITEM:	SERVING:
BREAKFAST		
152	POACHED EGGS	2 Large
185	Round Steak	3.75 oz.
70	Applesauce*	6 oz.
50	V8 Juice	8 oz.
68	Strawberries	1 Cup
525	**Breakfast Total**	
Snack 1		
50	Raspberries	1 Cup
100	Pudding (NS)	8 oz.
150	**Snack 1 Total**	
Lunch		
255	CHICKEN BRST (3)	7.5 oz.
40	Green SALAD	2 Cups
10	Mom's DRESSING	2 oz.
108	BBerries/StrawB	2 Cup
413	**Lunch Total**	
Snack 2		
120	Cottage Cheese	8 TBSP
55	Blackberries (NS)	1 Cups
175	**Snack 2 Total**	
Dinner		
370	Round STEAK (2)	3.75 oz.
30	Green SALAD	1.5 Cups
10	Mom's DRESSING	2 oz.
38	Peach Sliced	1 med
448	**Dinner Total**	
Snack 3		
50	Pudding (NS)	1/2 Large
40	BlueBerries	1/2 Cup
90	**Snack 2 Total**	

1801 TODAY'S Calorie TOTAL

© HCG DIET VICTORY
PLANNER.COM

'NO Sugar & Starch Diet Victory' EZPLAN™ — 1900 Calories

DATE: _____ **DATE:** _____ **DATE:** _____

Day 1

Record YOUR MORNING Weight: _____

✓	C:	ITEM:	SERVING:
		BREAKFAST	
○	152	POACHED EGGS	2 Large
○	185	Round Steak (1)	3.75 oz.
○	100	Applesauce	8 oz.
○	50	V8 Juice	8 oz.
○	60	Grapefruit	1/2
	547	**Breakfast Total**	
		Snack 1	
○	120	Cottage Cheese	8 TBSP
○	100	Tangerines	2 med
	220	**Snack 1 Total**	
		Lunch	
○	170	CHICKEN BRST (2)	7.5 oz.
○	50	Grn SALAD & Drsg	2 Cups
○	40	Blueberries	1 Cup
○	75	Apple Sliced	1 med
	335	**Lunch Total**	
		Snack 2	
○	100	Pudding (NS)	8 oz.
○	68	Strawberries (NS)	1 Cup
	168	**Snack 2 Total**	
		Dinner	
○	370	Round STEAK (2)	7.5 oz.
○	40	Spinach SLD/Drsg	1.5 Cups
○	38	Green Beans	1 Cup
○	100	Apple Sauce (NS)	8 oz.
	548	**Dinner Total**	
		Snack 3	
○	50	Pudding (NS)	7.5 oz.
○	40	BlueBerries	1 Cup
	90	**Snack 3 Total**	

1908 TODAY'S Calorie TOTAL

Day 2

Record YOUR MORNING Weight: _____

✓	C:	ITEM:	SERVING:
		BREAKFAST	
○	180	EGG Substitute	1 1/2 Cups
○	200	Chicken Sausage	2
○	100	Applesauce	8 oz.
○	40	Tomato Juice	4 oz.
○	60	Grapefruit	1/2
	580	**Breakfast Total**	
		Snack 1	
○	100	Pudding (NS)	8 oz.
○	40	BlueBerries	1 Cup
	140	**Snack 1 Total**	
		Lunch	
○	370	Round STEAK	7.5 oz.
○	40	Spinach SALAD	2 Cups
○	10	Mom's DRESSING	2 oz.
○	75	Apple Sliced	1 med
	495	**Lunch Total**	
		Snack 2	
○	120	Cottage Cheese	8 TBSP
○	68	Strawberries (NS)	1 Cups
	188	**Snack 2 Total**	
		Dinner	
○	170	CHICKEN BRST	7.5 oz.
○	40	Grn SALAD/Drsg	1.5 Cups
○	28	Cherry Tomatoes	1 Cup
○	100	Apple Sauce	8 oz.
	338	**Dinner Total**	
		Snack 3	
○	100	Pudding (NS)	8 oz.
○	55	Blackberries (NS)	1 Cup
	155	**Snack 2 Total**	

1896 TODAY'S Calorie TOTAL

Day 3

Record YOUR MORNING Weight: _____

✓	C:	ITEM:	SERVING:
		BREAKFAST	
○	228	POACHED EGGS	3 Large
○	40	BlueBerries	1 Cup
○	100	Applesauce	8 oz.
○	50	V8 Juice	8 oz.
○	68	Strawberries	1 Cup
	486	**Breakfast Total**	
		Snack 1	
○	50	Raspberries	1 Cup
○	100	Pudding (NS)	8 oz.
	150	**Snack 1 Total**	
		Lunch	
○	255	CHICKEN BRST (3)	11.25 oz.
○	50	Grn SALAD/Drsg	2 Cups
○	40	Blueberries	1 Cup
○	68	Strawberries (NS)	1 Cup
	413	**Lunch Total**	
		Snack 2	
○	120	Cottage Cheese	8 TBSP
○	55	Blackberries (NS)	1 Cups
	175	**Snack 2 Total**	
		Dinner	
○	370	Round STEAK (2)	7.5 oz.
○	40	Grn SALAD/Drsg	1.5 Cups
○	60	Grapefruit	1/2
○	76	Peach Sliced	2 med
	546	**Dinner Total**	
		Snack 3	
○	100	Pudding (NS)	8 oz.
○	40	BlueBerries	1 Cup
	140	**Snack 2 Total**	

1910 TODAY'S Calorie TOTAL

'NO Sugar & Starch Diet Victory' EZPLAN™   1900 Calories

DATE: 1900 — 4   Record YOUR MORNING Weight:

C:	ITEM:	SERVING:
BREAKFAST		
180	EGG Substitute	1 1/2 Cups
150	Pork Chop	3 oz.
70	Applesauce	6 oz.
50	V8 Juice	8 oz.
60	Grapefruit	1/2
510	**Breakfast Total**	
Snack 1		
120	Cottage Cheese	4 TBSP
40	BlueBerries	1 Cup
160	**Snack 1 Total**	
Lunch		
255	CHICKEN BRST (3)	11.25 oz.
50	Grn SALAD/Drsg	2 Cups
28	Black Berries	1/2 Cup
150	Apple Sliced	2 med
483	**Lunch Total**	
Snack 2		
100	Pudding (NS)	4 oz.
68	Strawberries (NS)	1 Cup
168	**Snack 2 Total**	
Dinner		
370	Round STEAK (2)	7.5 oz.
55	Black Berries	1 Cup
70	Apple Sauce (NS)	8 oz.
495	**Dinner Total**	
Snack 3		
50	Pudding (NS)	7.5 oz.
40	BlueBerries	1 Cup
90	**Snack 3 Total**	

1906   TODAY'S Calorie TOTAL

DATE: 1900 — 5   Record YOUR MORNING Weight:

C:	ITEM:	SERVING:
BREAKFAST		
228	POACHED EGGS	3 Large
100	Chicken Sausage	1
100	Applesauce*	8 oz.
40	Tomato Juice	8 oz.
60	Grapefruit	1/2
528	**Breakfast Total**	
Snack 1		
100	Pudding (NS)	4 oz.
60	BlueBerries	1 1/2 Cups
160	**Snack 1 Total**	
Lunch		
370	Round STEAK (2)	7.5 oz.
40	Spinach SALAD	2 Cups
10	Mom's DRESSING	2 oz.
75	Apple Sliced	1 med
495	**Lunch Total**	
Snack 2		
120	Cottage Cheese	8 TBSP
68	Strawberries (NS)	1 Cups
168	**Snack 2 Total**	
Dinner		
170	CHICKEN BRST (2)	7.5 oz.
40	Grn SALAD/Drsg	1.5 Cups
55	Blackberries	1 Cup
140	Apples Sliced	2 med
405	**Dinner Total**	
Snack 3		
100	Pudding (NS)	8 oz.
55	Blackberries (NS)	1 Cup
155	**Snack 2 Total**	

1911   TODAY'S Calorie TOTAL

DATE: 1900 — 6   Record YOUR MORNING Weight:

C:	ITEM:	SERVING:
BREAKFAST		
152	POACHED EGGS	2 Large
185	Round Steak	1/2 Cup
100	Applesauce*	8 oz.
50	V8 Juice	8 oz.
108	Sberries/BlueB	2 Cup
595	**Breakfast Total**	
Snack 1		
50	Raspberries	1 Cup
100	Pudding (NS)	4 oz.
150	**Snack 1 Total**	
Lunch		
255	CHICKEN BRST (3)	11.25 oz.
50	Grn SALAD/Drsg	2 Cups
40	Blueberries (NS)	1 Cup
34	Strawberries (NS)	1/2 Cup
379	**Lunch Total**	
Snack 2		
60	Cottage Cheese	4 TBSP
28	Blackberries (NS)	2 Cups
88	**Snack 2 Total**	
Dinner		
370	Round STEAK	7.5 oz.
40	Grn SALAD/Drsg	1.5 Cups
68	Strawberries (NS)	1 Cup
114	Peaches Sliced	3 med
592	**Dinner Total**	
Snack 3		
50	Pudding (NS)	1/2 Large
40	BlueBerries	1/2 Cup
90	**Snack 2 Total**	

1894   TODAY'S Calorie TOTAL

'NO Sugar & Starch Diet Victory' EZPLAN™ | 2000 Calories

Day 1

DATE: _____

2000 / 1 — Record YOUR MORNING Weight: _____

✓	C:	ITEM:	SERVING:
		BREAKFAST	
○	152	POACHED EGGS	2 Large
○	150	Lean Pork Chop	3 oz.
○	100	Applesauce	8 oz.
○	50	V8 Juice	8 oz.
○	60	Grapefruit	1/2
	512	Breakfast Total	
		Snack 1	
○	120	Cottage Cheese	8 TBSP
○	108	BlueB/SBerries	2 Cups
	228	Snack 1 Total	
		Lunch	
○	170	CHICKEN BRST(2)	7.5 oz.
○	50	Grn SALAD/Drsg	2 Cups
○	55	Blackberries	1 Cup
○	150	Apple Slices	2 med
	425	Lunch Total	
		Snack 2	
○	100	Pudding (NS)	8 oz.
○	102	Strawberries (NS)	1 1/2 Cups
	202	Snack 2 Total	
		Dinner	
○	370	Round STEAK (2)	7.5 oz.
○	40	Spin. SALAD/Drsg	2 Cups
○	38	Green Beans	1 Cup
○	100	Apple Sauce (NS)	8 oz.
	548	Dinner Total	
		Snack 3	
○	50	Pudding (NS)	7.5 oz.
○	40	BlueBerries	1 Cup
	90	Snack 3 Total	

2005 TODAY'S Calorie TOTAL

Day 2

DATE: _____

2000 / 2 — Record YOUR MORNING Weight: _____

✓	C:	ITEM:	SERVING:
		BREAKFAST	
○	152	POACHED EGG	2 Large
○	200	Chicken Sausage	2
○	100	Applesauce*	8 oz.
○	40	Tomato Juice	4 oz.
○	60	Grapefruit	1/2
	492	Breakfast Total	
		Snack 1	
○	100	Pudding (NS)	8 oz.
○	40	BlueBerries	1 Cup
	140	Snack 1 Total	
		Lunch	
○	370	Round STEAK (2)	7.5 oz.
○	50	Spin. SALAD	2 Cups
○	40	Blueberries	1 Cup
○	75	Apple Sliced	1 med
	535	Lunch Total	
		Snack 2	
○	120	Cottage Cheese	4 TBSP
○	68	Strawberries (NS)	1 Cups
	188	Snack 2 Total	
		Dinner	
○	255	CHICKEN BRST (3)	11.25 oz.
○	40	Grn. SALAD/Drsg	2 Cups
○	55	Strawberries	3/4 Cup
○	150	Apple Fresh Sliced	2 med
	500	Dinner Total	
		Snack 3	
○	100	Pudding (NS)	8 oz.
○	55	Blackberries (NS)	1/2 Cup
	155	Snack 2 Total	

2010 TODAY'S Calorie TOTAL

Day 3

DATE: _____

2000 / 3 — Record YOUR MORNING Weight: _____

✓	C:	ITEM:	SERVING:
		BREAKFAST	
○	152	POACHED EGGS	2 Large
○	185	Round Steak	3.75 oz
○	100	Applesauce	8 oz.
○	50	V8 Juice	8 oz.
○	34	Strawberries	1/2 Cup
	521	Breakfast Total	
		Snack 1	
○	75	Raspberries	1 1/2 Cups
○	100	Pudding (NS)	8 oz.
	175	Snack 1 Total	
		Lunch	
○	255	CHICKEN BRST (3)	11.25 oz.
○	50	Grn. SALAD/Drsg	2 Cups
○	50	Asparagus	8 oz.
○	68	Strawberries (NS)	1 Cup
	423	Lunch Total	
		Snack 2	
○	135	Cottage Cheese	9 TBSP
○	55	Blackberries (NS)	2 Cups
	190	Snack 2 Total	
		Dinner	
○	300	Lean P Chops (2)	3.75 oz.
○	40	Grn. SALAD/Drsg	2 Cups
○	100	Applesauce	8 oz.
○	76	Peach Slices	2 med
	516	Dinner Total	
		Snack 3	
○	100	Pudding (NS)	8 oz.
○	80	BlueBerries	2 Cups
	180	Snack 2 Total	

2005 TODAY'S Calorie TOTAL

'NO Sugar & Starch Diet Victory' EZPLAN™   2000 Calories

Day 4 (2000)

DATE:

Record YOUR MORNING Weight:

✓	C:	ITEM:	SERVING:
BREAKFAST			
○	180	Egg Substitute	1 1/2 Cups
○	150	Lean Pork Chop	1
○	100	Applesauce	8 oz.
○	50	V8 Juice	8 oz.
○	60	Grapefruit	1/2
	540	**Breakfast Total**	
Snack 1			
○	120	Cottage Cheese	8 TBSP
○	40	BlueBerries	1 Cup
	160	**Snack 1 Total**	
Lunch			
○	255	CHICKEN BRST(3)	11.25 oz.
○	50	Grn. SALAD/Drsg	2 Cups
○	38	Green Beans	1 Cup
○	150	Apple Sliced	2 med
	493	**Lunch Total**	
Snack 2			
○	100	Pudding (NS)	8 oz.
○	68	Strawberries (NS)	1 Cup
	168	**Snack 2 Total**	
Dinner			
○	370	Round STEAK (2)	7.5 oz.
○	40	Spin. SALAD/Drsg	2 Cups
○	44	Broccoli	1 Cup
○	100	Apple Sauce (NS)	8 oz.
	554	**Dinner Total**	
Snack 3			
○	50	Pudding (NS)	7.5 oz.
○	20	BlueBerries	1 Cup
	90	**Snack 3 Total**	

2005   TODAY'S Calorie TOTAL

Day 5 (2000)

DATE:

Record YOUR MORNING Weight:

✓	C:	ITEM:	SERVING:
BREAKFAST			
○	152	POACHED EGG	2 Large
○	185	Round Steak (1)	3.75 oz.
○	70	Applesauce	6 oz.
○	20	Tomato Juice	4 oz.
○	60	Grapefruit	1/2
	487	**Breakfast Total**	
Snack 1			
○	100	Pudding (NS)	4 oz.
○	80	BlueBerries	1 Cup
	180	**Snack 1 Total**	
Lunch			
○	255	Chicken BRST (3)	11.25 oz.
○	50	Spin. SALAD/Drsg	2 Cups
○	40	Blueberries	1 Cup
○	150	Apple Sliced	2 med
	495	**Lunch Total**	
Snack 2			
○	120	Cottage Cheese	8 TBSP
○	102	Strawberries (NS)	1 1/2 Cups
	222	**Snack 2 Total**	
Dinner			
○	300	Chick. Sausage (3)	2.3 0z
○	40	Grn. SALAD/Drsg	2 Cups
○	76	Green Beans	2 Cups
○	28	Cherry Tomatoes	1 Cup
	444	**Dinner Total**	
Snack 3			
○	100	Pudding (NS)	8 oz.
○	78	Blackberries (NS)	1 1/2 Cups
	178	**Snack 2 Total**	

2006   TODAY'S Calorie TOTAL

Day 6 (2000)

DATE:

Record YOUR MORNING Weight:

✓	C:	ITEM:	SERVING:
BREAKFAST			
○	152	POACHED EGGS	2 Large
○	136	Bacon Slices	4
○	100	Applesauce	8 oz.
○	40	Blueberries	1 Cup
○	68	Strawberries	1 Cup
	496	**Breakfast Total**	
Snack 1			
○	75	Raspberries	1 1/2 Cups
○	100	Pudding (NS)	8 oz.
	175	**Snack 1 Total**	
Lunch			
○	370	Round Steak (2)	7.5 oz.
○	50	Grn. SALAD/Drsg	2 Cups
○	40	Blueberries	2 oz.
○	68	Strawberries (NS)	1 Cup
	528	**Lunch Total**	
Snack 2			
○	120	Cottage Cheese	8 TBSP
○	110	Blackberries (NS)	1 1/2 Cups
	230	**Snack 2 Total**	
Dinner			
○	255	Chicken Breast	11.25 oz.
○	40	Grn. SALAD/Drsg	2 Cups
○	68	Strawberries	2 oz.
○	76	Peach Slices	2 med
	439	**Dinner Total**	
Snack 3			
○	100	Pudding (NS)	8 oz.
○	40	BlueBerries	1 1/2 Cups
	140	**Snack 2 Total**	

2008   TODAY'S Calorie TOTAL

'NO Sugar & Starch Diet Victory' EZPLAN™ | 2100 Calories

Day 1 — 2100

DATE:

Record YOUR MORNING Weight:

✓	C:	ITEM:	SERVING:
		BREAKFAST	
○	152	POACHED EGGS	2 Large
○	150	Ln Pork Chop (1)	3.75
○	100	Applesauce	8 oz.
○	50	V8 Juice	8 oz.
○	60	Grapefruit	1/2
	512	**Breakfast Total**	
		Snack 1	
○	120	Cottage Cheese	4 TBSP
○	108	BlueB/SBerries	2 Cup
	228	**Snack 1 Total**	
		Lunch	
○	170	CHICKEN BRST (2)	7.5 oz.
○	40	Grn. SALAD/Drsg	1 1/2 Cups
○	82	Blackberries	1 1/2 Cups
○	150	Apples Sliced	2 med
	452	**Lunch Total**	
		Snack 2	
○	100	Pudding (NS)	8 oz.
○	68	Strawberries (NS)	1 Cup
	168	**Snack 2 Total**	
		Dinner	
○	370	Round STEAK (2)	7.5 oz.
○	40	Spin. SALAD/Drsg	1.5 Cups
○	102	Strawberries	1 1/2 Cups
○	100	Apple Sauce (NS)	8 oz.
	612	**Dinner Total**	
		Snack 3	
○	100	Pudding (NS)	7.5 oz.
○	40	BlueBerries	1 Cup
	140	**Snack 3 Total**	

2102 TODAY'S Calorie TOTAL

Day 2 — 2100

DATE:

Record YOUR MORNING Weight:

✓	C:	ITEM:	SERVING:
		BREAKFAST	
○	180	EGG Substitute	2 Cups
○	200	Chicken Sausage	2
○	100	Applesauce	8 oz.
○	40	Tomato Juice	8 oz.
○	60	Grapefruit	1/2
	580	**Breakfast Total**	
		Snack 1	
○	100	Pudding (NS)	8 oz.
○	40	BlueBerries	1 Cup
	140	**Snack 1 Total**	
		Lunch	
○	370	Round STEAK (2)	7.5 oz.
○	50	Spin. SALAD/Drsg	2 Cups
○	80	Blueberries	2 Cups
○	150	Apples Sliced	2 med
	575	**Lunch Total**	
		Snack 2	
○	120	Cottage Cheese	8 TBSP
○	68	Strawberries (NS)	1 Cups
	188	**Snack 2 Total**	
		Dinner	
○	255	CHICKEN BRST (3)	11.25 oz.
○	40	Spin. SALAD	1.5 Cups
○	34	Strawberries	1/2 Cup
○	150	Apples Sliced	2 med
	479	**Dinner Total**	
		Snack 3	
○	100	Pudding (NS)	7.5 oz.
○	41	Blackberries (NS)	3/4 Cup
	141	**Snack 2 Total**	

2103 TODAY'S Calorie TOTAL

Day 3 — 2100

DATE:

Record YOUR MORNING Weight:

✓	C:	ITEM:	SERVING:
		BREAKFAST	
○	152	POACHED EGGS	2 Large
○	185	Round Steak (1)	1/2 Cup
○	100	Applesauce	8 oz.
○	50	V8 Juice	8 oz.
○	54	Sberries/BlueB	1/2 Cup
	541	**Breakfast Total**	
		Snack 1	
○	100	Raspberries	2 Cup
○	100	Pudding (NS)	8 oz.
	200	**Snack 1 Total**	
		Lunch	
○	255	CHICKEN BRST (3)	11.25 oz.
○	50	Grn. SALAD/Drsg	2 Cups
○	50	Asparagus	8 oz.
○	102	Strawberries (NS)	1 1/2 Cups
	457	**Lunch Total**	
		Snack 2	
○	135	Cottage Cheese	9 TBSP
○	83	Blackberries (NS)	1 1/2 Cups
	218	**Snack 2 Total**	
		Dinner	
○	300	Ln Pork Chops (2)	7.5 oz.
○	50	Grn. SALAD/Drsg	2 Cups
○	100	Applesauce	8 oz.
○	76	Peaches Sliced	2 med
	516	**Dinner Total**	
		Snack 3	
○	100	Pudding (NS)	8 oz.
○	60	BlueBerries	1 1/2 Cup
	160	**Snack 2 Total**	

2102 TODAY'S Calorie TOTAL

'NO Sugar & Starch Diet Victory' EZPLAN™ — 2100 Calories

Day 4 (2100)

DATE: _____   Record YOUR MORNING Weight: _____

✓	C:	ITEM:	SERVING:
		BREAKFAST	
○	180	EGG Substitute	2 Cups
○	150	Ln Pork Chop (1)	3 oz.
○	117	Applesauce	10 oz.
○	50	V8 Juice	8 oz.
○	60	Grapefruit	1/2
	557	**Breakfast Total**	
		Snack 1	
○	120	Cottage Cheese	8 TBSP
○	60	BlueBerries	1 1/2 Cup
	180	**Snack 1 Total**	
		Lunch	
○	255	CHICKEN BRST(3)	11.25 oz.
○	50	Grn. SALAD/Drsg	2 Cups
○	57	Green Beans	1 1/2 Cups
○	150	Apples Sliced	2 med
	512	**Lunch Total**	
		Snack 2	
○	100	Pudding (NS)	8 oz.
○	68	Strawberries (NS)	1 Cup
	168	**Snack 2 Total**	
		Dinner	
○	370	Round STEAK	7.5 oz.
○	40	Spin. SALAD/Drsg	1.5 Cups
○	44	Broccoli	1 Cup
○	117	Apple Sauce (NS)	10 oz.
	571	**Dinner Total**	
		Snack 3	
○	50	Pudding (NS)	7.5 oz.
○	60	BlueBerries	1 1/2 Cups
	110	**Snack 3 Total**	

2098 TODAY'S Calorie TOTAL

Day 5 (2100)

DATE: _____   Record YOUR MORNING Weight: _____

✓	C:	ITEM:	SERVING:
		BREAKFAST	
○	152	POACHED EGGS	2 Large
○	185	Round Steak (1)	3.75
○	100	Applesauce*	8 oz.
○	50	V-8 Juice	8 oz.
○	60	Grapefruit	1/2
	547	**Breakfast Total**	
		Snack 1	
○	100	Pudding (NS)	8 oz.
○	80	BlueBerries	2 Cups
	180	**Snack 1 Total**	
		Lunch	
○	255	CHICKEN BRST (2)	7.5 oz.
○	50	Spin. SALAD/Drsg	2 Cups
○	40	Blueberries	1 Cup
○	150	Apples Sliced	2 med
	495	**Lunch Total**	
		Snack 2	
○	120	Cottage Cheese	8 TBSP
○	102	Strawberries (NS)	1 1/2 Cups
	222	**Snack 2 Total**	
		Dinner	
○	300	Chicken Sausages	3
○	40	Grn. SALAD/Drsg	1.5 Cups
○	76	Green Beans	2 Cups
○	28	Cherry Tomatoes	1 Cup
	444	**Dinner Total**	
		Snack 3	
○	100	Pudding (NS)	7.5 oz.
○	110	Blackberries (NS)	1/2 Cup
	210	**Snack 2 Total**	

2098 TODAY'S Calorie TOTAL

Day 6 (2100)

DATE: _____   Record YOUR MORNING Weight: _____

✓	C:	ITEM:	SERVING:
		BREAKFAST	
○	228	POACHED EGGS	3 Large
○	130	Bacon Slices	4
○	100	Applesauce	8 oz.
○	40	Blueberries	8 oz.
○	68	Strawberries	1 Cup
	566	**Breakfast Total**	
		Snack 1	
○	75	Raspberries	1 1/2 Cups
○	100	Pudding (NS)	8 oz.
	175	**Snack 1 Total**	
		Lunch	
○	370	Round Steak (2)	7.5 oz.
○	50	Grn. SALAD/Drsg	2 Cups
○	60	Blueberries	1 1/2 Cups
○	68	Strawberries (NS)	1 Cup
	548	**Lunch Total**	
		Snack 2	
○	120	Cottage Cheese	8 TBSP
○	110	Blackberries (NS)	2 Cups
	230	**Snack 2 Total**	
		Dinner	
○	255	CHICKEN BRST (3)	11.25 oz.
○	40	Grn. SALAD/Drsg	1.5 Cups
○	55	Blackberries (NS)	1 cup
○	76	Peaches Sliced	2 med
	426	**Dinner Total**	
		Snack 3	
○	100	Pudding (NS)	1/2 Large
○	60	BlueBerries	1 1/2 Cups
	160	**Snack 2 Total**	

2105 TODAY'S Calorie TOTAL

'NO Sugar & Starch Diet Victory' EZPLAN™   2200 Calories

Day 1 — 2200

DATE:

Record YOUR MORNING Weight:

✓	C:	ITEM:	SERVING:
		BREAKFAST	
○	152	POACHED EGGs	2 Large
○	150	Lean Pork Chop	3 oz
○	117	Applesauce	10 oz.
○	50	V8 Juice	8 oz.
○	60	Grapefruit	1/2
	529	**Breakfast Total**	
		Snack 1	
○	120	Cottage Cheese	8 TBSP
○	108	BlueB/SBerries	2 Cup
	228	**Snack 1 Total**	
		Lunch	
○	170	CHICKEN BRST(2)	7.5 oz.
○	50	Grn. SALAD/Drsg	2 Cups
○	110	Blackberries	2 Cups
○	150	Apple Sliced	2 med
	480	**Lunch Total**	
		Snack 2	
○	100	Pudding (NS)	8 oz.
○	68	Strawberries (NS)	1 Cup
	168	**Snack 2 Total**	
		Dinner	
○	370	Round STEAK (2)	7.5 oz.
○	50	Spin. SALAD/Drsg	2 Cups
○	136	Strawberries	2 Cups
○	117	Apple Sauce (NS)	10 oz.
	673	**Dinner Total**	
		Snack 3	
○	100	Pudding (NS)	7.5 oz.
○	20	BlueBerries	1/2 Cup
	120	**Snack 3 Total**	

2198 TODAY'S Calorie TOTAL

Day 2 — 2200

DATE:

Record YOUR MORNING Weight:

✓	C:	ITEM:	SERVING:
		BREAKFAST	
○	180	EGG Substitute	2 Cups
○	200	Chicken Sausage	2
○	117	Applesauce	10 oz.
○	40	Tomato Juice	8 oz.
○	60	Grapefruit	1/2
	597	**Breakfast Total**	
		Snack 1	
○	100	Pudding (NS)	8 oz.
○	40	BlueBerries	1 Cup
	140	**Snack 1 Total**	
		Lunch	
○	370	Round STEAK (2)	7.5 oz.
○	50	Spin. SALAD/Drsg	2 Cups
○	80	Blueberries	2 Cups
○	150	Apple Sliced	2 med
	650	**Lunch Total**	
		Snack 2	
○	120	Cottage Cheese	8 TBSP
○	68	Strawberries (NS)	1 Cups
	188	**Snack 2 Total**	
		Dinner	
○	255	CHICKEN BRST (3)	11.25 oz.
○	50	Grn. SALAD/Drsg	2 Cups
○	41	Blackberries	3/4 Cup
○	150	Apple Fresh Sliced	2 med
	496	**Dinner Total**	
		Snack 3	
○	100	Pudding (NS)	8 oz.
○	28	Blackberries (NS)	1/2 Cup
	128	**Snack 2 Total**	

2199 TODAY'S Calorie TOTAL

Day 3 — 2200

DATE:

Record YOUR MORNING Weight:

✓	C:	ITEM:	SERVING:
		BREAKFAST	
○	152	POACHED EGGS	2 Large
○	185	Round Steak (1)	3.75 oz.
○	117	Applesauce	10 oz.
○	50	V8 Juice	8 oz.
○	81	Sberries/BlueB	1 1/2 Cups
	585	**Breakfast Total**	
		Snack 1	
○	100	Raspberries	2 Cup
○	100	Pudding (NS)	8 oz.
	200	**Snack 1 Total**	
		Lunch	
○	255	CHICKEN BRST (3)	11.25 oz.
○	50	Grn. SALAD/Drsg	2 Cups
○	75	Asparagus	12 oz.
○	102	Strawberries (NS)	1 1/2 Cup
	482	**Lunch Total**	
		Snack 2	
○	135	Cottage Cheese	8 TBSP
○	110	Blackberries (NS)	2 Cups
	245	**Snack 2 Total**	
		Dinner	
○	300	Ln. Pork Chops (2)	6 oz.
○	50	Grn. SALAD/Drsg	2 Cups
○	117	Applesauce	10 oz.
○	76	Peaches Sliced	2 med
	543	**Dinner Total**	
		Snack 3	
○	100	Pudding (NS)	8 oz.
○	40	BlueBerries	1 Cup
	140	**Snack 2 Total**	

2195 TODAY'S Calorie TOTAL

'NO Sugar & Starch Diet Victory' EZPLAN™ | 2200 Calories

DAY 4 — 2200

DATE: _____

Record YOUR MORNING Weight: _____

✓	C:	ITEM:	SERVING:
		BREAKFAST	
○	180	EGG Substitute	2 Cups
○	150	Ln. Pork Chop	3 oz.
○	140	Applesauce	12 oz.
○	50	V8 Juice	8 oz.
○	60	Grapefruit	1/2
	580	**Breakfast Total**	
		Snack 1	
○	120	Cottage Cheese	8 TBSP
○	60	BlueBerries	1 1/2 Cup
	180	**Snack 1 Total**	
		Lunch	
○	255	CHICKEN BRST (3)	11.25 oz.
○	50	Grn. SALAD/Drsg	2 Cups
○	76	Green Beans	2 Cups
○	150	Apples Sliced	2 med
	531	**Lunch Total**	
		Snack 2	
○	100	Pudding (NS)	8 oz.
○	68	Strawberries (NS)	1 Cup
	168	**Snack 2 Total**	
		Dinner	
○	370	Round STEAK (2)	3.75 oz.
○	50	Spin. SALAD/Drsg	2 Cups
○	44	Broccoli	1 Cup
○	140	Apple Sauce (NS)	12 oz.
	604	**Dinner Total**	
		Snack 3	
○	100	Pudding (NS)	8 oz.
○	40	BlueBerries	1 Cup
	140	**Snack 3 Total**	

2203 TODAY'S Calorie TOTAL

DAY 5 — 2200

DATE: _____

Record YOUR MORNING Weight: _____

✓	C:	ITEM:	SERVING:
		BREAKFAST	
○	152	POACHED EGGS	2 Large
○	185	Round STEAK	3.75 oz.
○	140	Applesauce	12 oz.
○	40	Tomato Juice	8 oz.
○	60	Grapefruit	1/2
	577	**Breakfast Total**	
		Snack 1	
○	100	Pudding (NS)	8 oz.
○	80	BlueBerries	2 Cup
	180	**Snack 1 Total**	
		Lunch	
○	255	CHICKEN BRST (3)	11.25 oz.
○	50	Spin. SALAD/Drsg	2 Cups
○	108	SBerries/BlueB	2 cups
○	150	Apple Sliced	2 med
	563	**Lunch Total**	
		Snack 2	
○	120	Cottage Cheese	8 TBSP
○	102	Strawberries (NS)	1 1/2 Cups
	222	**Snack 2 Total**	
		Dinner	
○	300	Chicken Sausages	3
○	40	Grn. SALAD/Drsg	1 1/2 Cups
○	76	Green Beans	2 Cups.
○	28	Cherry Tomatoes	1 Cup
	444	**Dinner Total**	
		Snack 3	
○	100	Pudding (NS)	7.5 oz.
○	110	Blackberries (NS)	2 Cups
	220	**Snack 2 Total**	

2206 TODAY'S Calorie TOTAL

DAY 6 — 2200

DATE: _____

Record YOUR MORNING Weight: _____

✓	C:	ITEM:	SERVING:
		BREAKFAST	
○	228	POACHED EGGS	3 Large
○	200	Chicken Sausages	2
○	140	Applesauce	12 oz.
○	50	V8 Juice	8 oz.
○	34	Strawberries	1/2 Cup
	652	**Breakfast Total**	
		Snack 1	
○	75	Raspberries	1 Cup
○	100	Pudding (NS)	4 oz.
	175	**Snack 1 Total**	
		Lunch	
○	370	Round Steak (2)	7.5 oz.
○	50	Grn. SALAD/Drsg	2 Cups
○	60	Blueberries	1 1/2 Cups
○	68	Strawberries (NS)	1 Cup
	548	**Lunch Total**	
		Snack 2	
○	120	Cottage Cheese	8 TBSP
○	55	Blackberries (NS)	2 Cups
	175	**Snack 2 Total**	
		Dinner	
○	255	Chicken BRST (3)	11.25 oz.
○	50	Grn. SALAD/Drsg	2 Cups
○	80	Blueberries	2 Cups
○	76	Peach Sliced	2 med
	465	**Dinner Total**	
		Snack 3	
○	100	Pudding (NS)	8 oz.
○	82	BlackBerries	1 1/2 Cup
	182	**Snack 2 Total**	

2197 TODAY'S Calorie TOTAL

'NO Sugar & Starch Diet Victory' EZPLAN™ | 2300 Calories

DATE: _____   DATE: _____   DATE: _____

2300 — 1   Record YOUR MORNING Weight: _____

✓	C:	ITEM:	SERVING:
		BREAKFAST	
○	228	POACHED EGGS	3 Large
○	150	Lean Pork Chop	3 oz.
○	117	Applesauce	10 oz.
○	50	V8 Juice	8 oz.
○	60	Grapefruit	1/2
	605	**Breakfast Total**	
		Snack 1	
○	120	Cottage Cheese	8 TBSP
○	60	BlueBerries	1 1/2 Cup
	180	**Snack 1 Total**	
		Lunch	
○	170	CHICKEN BRST (2)	7.5 oz.
○	50	Grn. SALAD/Drsg	2 Cups
○	110	Blackberries	2 Cups
○	150	Apples Sliced	2 med
	480	**Lunch Total**	
		Snack 2	
○	100	Pudding (NS)	8 oz.
○	102	Strawberries (NS)	1 1/2 Cups
	202	**Snack 2 Total**	
		Dinner	
○	370	Round STEAK (2)	7.5 oz.
○	40	Spin. SALAD/Drsg	1.5 Cups
○	108	Strawberries	1 1/2 Cups
○	140	Apple Sauce (NS)	12 oz.
	658	**Dinner Total**	
		Snack 3	
○	100	Pudding (NS)	8 oz.
○	80	BlueBerries	2 Cup
	180	**Snack 3 Total**	

2305 TODAY'S Calorie TOTAL

2300 — 2   Record YOUR MORNING Weight: _____

✓	C:	ITEM:	SERVING:
		BREAKFAST	
○	180	EGG Substitute	2 Cups
○	300	Chicken Sausages	3
○	117	Applesauce	10 oz.
○	40	Tomato Juice	8 oz.
○	60	Grapefruit	1/2
	697	**Breakfast Total**	
		Snack 1	
○	100	Pudding (NS)	4 oz.
○	40	BlueBerries	1 Cup
	140	**Snack 1 Total**	
		Lunch	
○	370	Round STEAK (2)	7.5 oz.
○	50	Spin. SALAD/Drsg	2 Cups
○	80	Blueberries	2 Cups
○	150	Apples Sliced	2 med
	650	**Lunch Total**	
		Snack 2	
○	120	Cottage Cheese	8 TBSP
○	68	Strawberries (NS)	1 Cup
	188	**Snack 2 Total**	
		Dinner	
○	255	CHICKEN BRST (3)	11.25 oz.
○	50	Grn. SALAD/Drsg	2 Cups
○	41	Blackberries	3/4 Cup
○	150	Apples Sliced	2 med
	496	**Dinner Total**	
		Snack 3	
○	100	Pudding (NS)	8 oz.
○	28	Blackberries (NS)	1/2 Cup
	128	**Snack 2 Total**	

2299 TODAY'S Calorie TOTAL

2300 — 3   Record YOUR MORNING Weight: _____

✓	C:	ITEM:	SERVING:
		BREAKFAST	
○	228	POACHED EGGS	3 Large
○	185	Round Steak	3.75 oz.
○	117	Applesauce	10 oz.
○	50	V8 Juice	8 oz.
○	108	Sberries/BlueB	2 Cups
	688	**Breakfast Total**	
		Snack 1	
○	100	Raspberries	2 Cup
○	100	Pudding (NS)	8 oz.
	200	**Snack 1 Total**	
		Lunch	
○	255	CHICKEN BRST (3)	11.25 oz.
○	50	Grn. SALAD/Drsg	2 Cups
○	75	Asparagus	12 oz.
○	102	Strawberries (NS)	1 1/2 Cup
	482	**Lunch Total**	
		Snack 2	
○	135	Cottage Cheese	9 TBSP
○	110	Blackberries (NS)	2 Cups
	245	**Snack 2 Total**	
		Dinner	
○	300	Lean P. Chops (2)	7.5 oz.
○	50	Grn. SALAD/Drsg	2 Cups
○	117	Applesauce (NS)	10 oz.
○	76	Peaches Sliced	2 med
	543	**Dinner Total**	
		Snack 3	
○	100	Pudding (NS)	8 oz.
○	40	BlueBerries	1 Cup
	140	**Snack 2 Total**	

2298 TODAY'S Calorie TOTAL

'NO Sugar & Starch Diet Victory' EZPLAN™ | 2300 Calories

DAY 4

DATE:

2300 — 4

Record YOUR MORNING Weight:

✓	C:	ITEM:	SERVING:
		BREAKFAST	
○	225	EGG Substitute	2 1/2 Cups
○	150	Lean P. Chop (1)	3 oz.
○	140	Applesauce	12 oz.
○	50	V8 Juice	8 oz.
○	60	Grapefruit	1/2
	625	Breakfast Total	
		Snack 1	
○	120	Cottage Cheese	8 TBSP
○	60	BlueBerries	1 1/2 Cups
	180	Snack 1 Total	
		Lunch	
○	255	CHICKEN BRST (3)	11.25 oz.
○	50	Grn. SALAD/Drsg	2 Cups
○	76	Green Beans	2 Cups
○	150	Apples Sliced	2 med
	531	Lunch Total	
		Snack 2	
○	100	Pudding (NS)	8 oz.
○	136	Strawberries (NS)	2 Cup
	236	Snack 2 Total	
		Dinner	
○	370	Round STEAK (2)	7.5 oz.
○	40	Spin. SALAD/Drsg	1.5 Cups
○	44	Broccoli	1 Cup
○	140	Apple Sauce (NS)	12 oz.
	594	Dinner Total	
		Snack 3	
○	100	Pudding (NS)	8 oz.
○	40	BlueBerries	1 Cup
	140	Snack 3 Total	

2306 TODAY'S Calorie TOTAL

DAY 5

DATE:

2300 — 5

Record YOUR MORNING Weight:

✓	C:	ITEM:	SERVING:
		BREAKFAST	
○	228	POACHED EGGS	3 Large
○	200	Chicken Sausages	2
○	140	Applesauce	12 oz.
○	40	Tomato Juice	8 oz.
○	60	Grapefruit	1/2
	668	Breakfast Total	
		Snack 1	
○	100	Pudding (NS)	8 oz.
○	80	BlueBerries	2 Cup
	180	Snack 1 Total	
		Lunch	
○	255	Chcken BRST (3)	11.25 oz.
○	40	Spin. SALAD/Drsg	1 1/2 Cups
○	108	SBerries/BlueB	2 Cups
○	150	Apple Sliced	2 med
	553	Lunch Total	
		Snack 2	
○	120	Cottage Cheese	8 TBSP
○	102	Strawberries (NS)	1 1/2 Cups
	222	Snack 2 Total	
		Dinner	
○	300	Lean P. Chops (2)	6 oz.
○	40	Green SALAD	1.5 Cups
○	57	Green Beans	1 1/2 Cups
○	150	Apples Sliced	2 med
	547	Dinner Total	
		Snack 3	
○	100	Pudding (NS)	7.5 oz.
○	28	Blackberries (NS)	1/2 Cup
	128	Snack 2 Total	

2298 TODAY'S Calorie TOTAL

DAY 6

DATE:

2300 — 6

Record YOUR MORNING Weight:

✓	C:	ITEM:	SERVING:
		BREAKFAST	
○	228	POACHED EGGS	3 Large
○	300	Chicken Sausages	3
○	140	Applesauce	12 oz.
○	50	V8 Juice	8 oz.
○	34	Strawberries	1/2 Cup
	752	Breakfast Total	
		Snack 1	
○	75	Raspberries	1 1/2 Cups
○	100	Pudding (NS)	8 oz.
	175	Snack 1 Total	
		Lunch	
○	370	Round Steak (2)	7.5 oz.
○	50	Grn. SALAD/Drsg	2 Cups
○	60	Blueberries	1 1/2 Cups
○	68	Strawberries (NS)	1 Cup
	548	Lunch Total	
		Snack 2	
○	120	Cottage Cheese	8 TBSP
○	55	Blackberries (NS)	1 Cup
	175	Snack 2 Total	
		Dinner	
○	255	Chicken BRST (3)	11.25 oz.
○	50	Grn. SALAD/Drsg	2 Cups
○	80	Blueberries	2 Cups
○	76	Peaches Sliced	2 med
	461	Dinner Total	
		Snack 3	
○	100	Pudding (NS)	8 oz.
○	80	BlueBerries	2 Cup
	180	Snack 2 Total	

2291 TODAY'S Calorie TOTAL

'NO Sugar & Starch Diet Victory' EZPLAN™   2400 Calories

Day 1

DATE:

2400 / 1

Record YOUR MORNING Weight:

✓	C:	ITEM:	SERVING:
		BREAKFAST	
○	225	POACHED EGGs	3 Large
○	150	Lean P. CHOP	1
○	140	Applesauce	12 oz.
○	50	V8 Juice	8 oz.
○	60	Grapefruit	1/2
	628	**Breakfast Total**	
		Snack 1	
○	150	Cottage Cheese	10 TBSP
○	80	BlueBerries	2 Cup
	230	**Snack 1 Total**	
		Lunch	
○	170	CHICKEN BRST (2)	7.5 oz.
○	50	Grn. SALAD/Drsg	2 Cups
○	110	Blackberries	2 Cups
○	150	Apples Sliced	2 med
	480	**Lunch Total**	
		Snack 2	
○	100	Pudding (NS)	8 oz.
○	136	Strawberries (NS)	2 Cups
	236	**Snack 2 Total**	
		Dinner	
○	370	Round STEAK (2)	7.5 oz.
○	50	Spin. SALAD/Drsg	2 Cups
○	162	SBerries/BlueB	3 Cups
○	117	Apple Sauce (NS)	10 oz.
	699	**Dinner Total**	
		Snack 3	
○	100	Pudding (NS)	8 oz.
○	30	BlueBerries	3/4 Cup
	130	**Snack 3 Total**	

2403   TODAY'S Calorie TOTAL

Day 2

DATE:

2400 / 2

Record YOUR MORNING Weight:

✓	C:	ITEM:	SERVING:
		BREAKFAST	
○	228	POACHED EGGs	3 Large
○	300	Chicken Sausages	3
○	117	Applesauce	10 oz.
○	40	Tomato Juice	8 oz.
○	60	Grapefruit	1/2
	745	**Breakfast Total**	
		Snack 1	
○	100	Pudding (NS)	4 oz.
○	82	BlackBerries	1 1/2 Cups
	182	**Snack 1 Total**	
		Lunch	
○	370	Round STEAK (2)	7.5 oz.
○	50	Spin. SALAD/Drsg	2 Cups
○	80	Blueberries	2 Cups
○	150	Apple Sliced	2 med
	650	**Lunch Total**	
		Snack 2	
○	120	Cottage Cheese	8 TBSP
○	68	Strawberries (NS)	1 Cups
	188	**Snack 2 Total**	
		Dinner	
○	255	CHICKEN BRST (3)	11.25 oz.
○	50	Grn. SALAD/Drsg	2 Cups
○	41	Blackberries	3/4 Cup
○	150	Apples Sliced	2 med
	496	**Dinner Total**	
		Snack 3	
○	100	Pudding (NS)	8 oz.
○	40	Blackberries (NS)	1 Cup
	140	**Snack 2 Total**	

2401   TODAY'S Calorie TOTAL

Day 3

DATE:

2400 / 3

Record YOUR MORNING Weight:

✓	C:	ITEM:	SERVING:
		BREAKFAST	
○	228	POACHED EGGs	3 Large
○	185	Round Steak	3.75 oz.
○	117	Applesauce	10 oz.
○	50	V8 Juice	8 oz.
○	162	Sberries/BlueB	3 Cups
	742	**Breakfast Total**	
		Snack 1	
○	100	Raspberries	2 Cup
○	100	Pudding (NS)	8 oz.
	200	**Snack 1 Total**	
		Lunch	
○	255	CHICKEN BRST (3)	11.25 oz.
○	50	Grn. SALAD/Drsg	2 Cups
○	75	Asparagus	12 oz.
○	136	Strawberries (NS)	2 Cup
	516	**Lunch Total**	
		Snack 2	
○	150	Cottage Cheese	10 TBSP
○	110	Blackberries (NS)	2 Cups
	260	**Snack 2 Total**	
		Dinner	
○	300	Lean P. CHOPS (2)	6 oz.
○	50	Grn. SALAD/Drsg	2 Cups
○	117	Applesauce (NS)	10 oz.
○	76	Peaches Sliced	2 med
	543	**Dinner Total**	
		Snack 3	
○	100	Pudding (NS)	8 oz.
○	40	BlueBerries	1 Cup
	140	**Snack 2 Total**	

2401   TODAY'S Calorie TOTAL

'NO Sugar & Starch Diet Victory' EZPLAN™   2400 Calories

DATE: **DATE:**   **DATE:**

Day 4 (2400) — Record YOUR MORNING Weight:

✓	C:	ITEM:	SERVING:
BREAKFAST			
○	220	EGG Substitute	3 Cups
○	150	Lean P.CHOP (1)	3 oz.
○	140	Applesauce	12 oz.
○	50	V8 Juice	8 oz.
○	60	Grapefruit	1/2
	620	Breakfast Total	
Snack 1			
○	140	Cottage Cheese	10 TBSP
○	80	BlueBerries	2 Cup
	220	Snack 1 Total	
Lunch			
○	255	CHICKEN BRST(2)	7.5 oz.
○	50	Grn. SALAD/Drsg	2 Cups
○	76	Green Beans	2 Cups
○	150	Apple Sliced	2 med
	531	Lunch Total	
Snack 2			
○	100	Pudding (NS)	8 oz.
○	136	Strawberries (NS)	2 Cups
	236	Snack 2 Total	
Dinner			
○	370	Round STEAK (2)	7.5 oz.
○	50	Spin. SALAD/Drsg	2 Cups
○	88	Broccoli	2 Cups
○	140	Apple Sauce (NS)	12 oz.
	648	Dinner Total	
Snack 3			
○	100	Pudding (NS)	8 oz.
○	40	BlueBerries	1 Cup
	140	Snack 3 Total	

2395 — TODAY'S Calorie TOTAL

Day 5 (2400) — Record YOUR MORNING Weight:

✓	C:	ITEM:	SERVING:
BREAKFAST			
○	228	POACHED EGG	3 Large
○	300	Chicken Sausage	3
○	140	Applesauce	12 oz.
○	40	Tomato Juice	8 oz.
○	60	Grapefruit	1/2
	768	Breakfast Total	
Snack 1			
○	100	Pudding (NS)	8 oz.
○	80	BlueBerries	2 Cup
	180	Snack 1 Total	
Lunch			
○	255	Chicken BRST (3)	11.25 oz.
○	40	Spin. SALAD/Drsg	1 1/2 Cups
○	108	SBerries/BlueB	2 Cups
○	150	Apple Sliced	1 med
	553	Lunch Total	
Snack 2			
○	120	Cottage Cheese	8 TBSP
○	102	SBerries/BlueB	1 1/2 Cups
	222	Snack 2 Total	
Dinner			
○	300	Lean P.CHOP (2)	6 oz.
○	40	Grn. SALAD/Drsg	1.5 Cups
○	57	Green Beans	1 1/2 Cups
○	150	Apples Sliced	2 med
	547	Dinner Total	
Snack 3			
○	100	Pudding (NS)	8 oz.
○	28	Blackberries (NS)	1/2 Cup
	128	Snack 2 Total	

2398 — TODAY'S Calorie TOTAL

Day 6 (2400) — Record YOUR MORNING Weight:

✓	C:	ITEM:	SERVING:
BREAKFAST			
○	228	POACHED EGGS	3 Large
○	300	Chicken Sausages	3
○	140	Applesauce	12 oz.
○	50	V8 Juice	8 oz.
○	34	Strawberries	1/2 Cup
	752	Breakfast Total	
Snack 1			
○	100	Raspberries	2 Cup
○	100	Pudding (NS)	8 oz.
	200	Snack 1 Total	
Lunch			
○	370	Round Steak (2)	7.5 oz.
○	50	Grn. SALAD/Drsg	2 Cups
○	80	Blueberries	2 Cups
○	68	Strawberries (NS)	1 Cup
	568	Lunch Total	
Snack 2			
○	120	Cottage Cheese	8 TBSP
○	110	Blackberries (NS)	2 Cups
	230	Snack 2 Total	
Dinner			
○	255	Chicken BRST (3)	11.25 oz.
○	50	Grn. SALAD/Drsg	2 Cups
○	80	Blueberries	2 Cups
○	76	Peaches Sliced	2 med
	461	Dinner Total	
Snack 3			
○	100	Pudding (NS)	8 oz.
○	80	BlueBerries	2 Cups
	180	Snack 2 Total	

2391 — TODAY'S Calorie TOTAL

'NO Sugar & Starch Diet Victory' EZPLAN™   2500 Calories

Day 1 — 2500

DATE:

Record YOUR MORNING Weight:

✓	C:	ITEM:	SERVING:
BREAKFAST			
○	152	POACHED EGGS	2 Large
○	300	Lean P. CHOPS (2)	6 oz.
○	140	Applesauce	12 oz.
○	50	V8 Juice	8 oz.
○	60	Grapefruit	1/2
	702	**Breakfast Total**	
Snack 1			
○	150	Cottage Cheese	10 TBSP
○	80	Blueberries	2 Cups
	230	**Snack 1 Total**	
Lunch			
○	170	CHICKEN BRST (2)	7.5 oz.
○	50	Grn. SALAD/Drsg	2 Cups
○	110	Blackberries	2 Cups
○	150	Apples Sliced	2 med
	480	**Lunch Total**	
Snack 2			
○	100	Pudding (NS)	8 oz.
○	136	Strawberries (NS)	2 Cups
	236	**Snack 2 Total**	
Dinner			
○	370	Round STEAK (2)	7.5 oz.
○	50	Spin. SALAD/Drsg	2 Cups
○	162	SBerries/BlueB	3 Cups
○	140	Apple Sauce (NS)	12 oz.
	722	**Dinner Total**	
Snack 3			
○	100	Pudding (NS)	8 oz.
○	30	BlueBerries	3/4 Cup
	130	**Snack 3 Total**	
2500		**TODAY'S Calorie TOTAL**	

Day 2 — 2500

DATE:

Record YOUR MORNING Weight:

✓	C:	ITEM:	SERVING:
BREAKFAST			
○	228	POACHED EGGS	3 Large
○	300	Chicken Sausage	3
○	140	Applesauce	12 oz.
○	20	Tomato Juice	4 oz.
○	120	Grapefruit	1 med
	808	**Breakfast Total**	
Snack 1			
○	100	Pudding (NS)	8 oz.
○	110	Blackberries	2 Cup
	210	**Snack 1 Total**	
Lunch			
○	370	Round STEAK (2)	7.5 oz.
○	50	Spin. SALAD/Drsg	2 Cups
○	108	SBerries/BlueB	2 Cups
○	150	Apple Sliced	2 med
	678	**Lunch Total**	
Snack 2			
○	135	Cottage Cheese	9 TBSP
○	68	Strawberries (NS)	1 Cups
	203	**Snack 2 Total**	
Dinner			
○	255	CHICKEN BRST (3)	11.25 oz.
○	50	Grn. SALAD/Drsg	2 Cups
○	26	Blackberries	1/2 Cup
○	150	Apple Fresh Sliced	2 med
	481	**Dinner Total**	
Snack 3			
○	100	Pudding (NS)	8 oz.
○	20	Blueberries (NS)	1/2 Cup
	120	**Snack 2 Total**	
2500		**TODAY'S Calorie TOTAL**	

Day 3 — 2500

DATE:

Record YOUR MORNING Weight:

✓	C:	ITEM:	SERVING:
BREAKFAST			
○	152	POACHED EGGS	2 Large
○	370	Round Steak (2)	7.5 oz.
○	117	Applesauce*	10 oz.
○	50	V8 Juice	8 oz.
○	135	SBerries/BlueB	2 1/2 Cups
	824	**Breakfast Total**	
Snack 1			
○	100	Raspberries	2 Cups
○	100	Pudding (NS)	8 oz.
	200	**Snack 1 Total**	
Lunch			
○	255	CHICKEN BRST (3)	11.25 oz.
○	50	Grn. SALAD/Drsg	2 Cups
○	75	Asparagus	12 oz.
○	136	Strawberries (NS)	2 Cups
	516	**Lunch Total**	
Snack 2			
○	150	Cottage Cheese	10 TBSP
○	110	Blackberries (NS)	2 Cups
	260	**Snack 2 Total**	
Dinner			
○	300	Lean P. CHOPS (2)	6 oz.
○	50	Grn. SALAD/Drsg	2 Cups
○	140	Applesauce (NS)	12 oz.
○	76	Peaches Sliced	2 med
	566	**Dinner Total**	
Snack 3			
○	100	Pudding (NS)	8 oz.
○	40	BlueBerries	1 Cup
	140	**Snack 2 Total**	
2506		**TODAY'S Calorie TOTAL**	

'NO Sugar & Starch Diet Victory' EZPLAN™ | 2500 Calories

DAY 4

DATE: _____

2500 — 4

Record YOUR MORNING Weight: _____

✓	C:	ITEM:	SERVING:
		BREAKFAST	
○	220	EGG Substitute	3 Cups
○	300	Lean P CHOP (2)	6 oz.
○	140	Applesauce	12 oz.
○	50	V8 Juice	8 oz.
○	60	Grapefruit	1/2
	770	**Breakfast Total**	
		Snack 1	
○	120	Cottage Cheese	8 TBSP
○	80	BlueBerries	2 Cup
	200	**Snack 1 Total**	
		Lunch	
○	255	CHICKEN BRST (3)	11.25 oz.
○	50	Grn. SALAD/Drsg	2 Cups
○	76	Green Beans	2 Cups
○	150	Apples Sliced	2 med
	531	**Lunch Total**	
		Snack 2	
○	100	Pudding (NS)	8 oz.
○	136	Strawberries (NS)	2 Cups
	236	**Snack 2 Total**	
		Dinner	
○	370	Round STEAK (2)	7.5 oz.
○	50	Spin. SALAD/Drsg	2 Cups
○	88	Broccoli	2 Cups
○	140	Apple Sauce (NS)	12 oz.
	648	**Dinner Total**	
		Snack 3	
○	100	Pudding (NS)	7.5 oz.
○	20	BlueBerries	1/2 Cup
	120	**Snack 3 Total**	

2505 — TODAY'S Calorie TOTAL

DAY 5

DATE: _____

2500 — 5

Record YOUR MORNING Weight: _____

✓	C:	ITEM:	SERVING:
		BREAKFAST	
○	228	POACHED EGGS	3 Large
○	400	Chicken Sausages	4
○	140	Applesauce	12 oz.
○	40	Tomato Juice	8 oz.
○	60	Grapefruit	1/2
	868	**Breakfast Total**	
		Snack 1	
○	100	Pudding (NS)	8 oz.
○	80	BlueBerries	2 Cups
	180	**Snack 1 Total**	
		Lunch	
○	255	Chicken BRST (3)	11.25 oz.
○	40	Spin. SALAD/Drsg	1 1/2 Cups
○	108	SBerries/BlueB	2 Cups
○	150	Apples Sliced	2 med
	553	**Lunch Total**	
		Snack 2	
○	120	Cottage Cheese	8 TBSP
○	108	SBerries/BlueB	2 Cups
	228	**Snack 2 Total**	
		Dinner	
○	300	Lean P. CHOPS (2)	6 oz.
○	40	Grn. SALAD/Drsg	1.5 Cups
○	57	Green Beans	1 1/2 Cups
○	150	Apples Sliced	2 med
	547	**Dinner Total**	
		Snack 3	
○	100	Pudding (NS)	7.5 oz.
○	28	Blackberries (NS)	1/2 Cup
	128	**Snack 2 Total**	

2504 — TODAY'S Calorie TOTAL

DAY 6

DATE: _____

2500 — 6

Record YOUR MORNING Weight: _____

✓	C:	ITEM:	SERVING:
		BREAKFAST	
○	228	POACHED EGGS	3 Large
○	400	Chicken Sausages	4
○	140	Applesauce	12 oz.
○	50	V8 Juice	8 oz.
○	51	Strawberries	3/4 Cup
	869	**Breakfast Total**	
		Snack 1	
○	100	Raspberries	2 Cup
○	100	Pudding (NS)	8 oz.
	200	**Snack 1 Total**	
		Lunch	
○	370	Round STEAK (2)	7.5 oz.
○	50	Grn. SALAD/Drsg	2 Cups
○	80	Blueberries	2 Cups
○	68	Strawberries (NS)	1 Cup
	568	**Lunch Total**	
		Snack 2	
○	120	Cottage Cheese	8 TBSP
○	110	Blackberries (NS)	2 Cups
	230	**Snack 2 Total**	
		Dinner	
○	255	Chicken BRST (3)	11.25 oz.
○	50	Grn. SALAD/Drsg	2 Cups
○	80	Blueberries	2 Cups
○	76	Peaches Sliced	2 med
	461	**Dinner Total**	
		Snack 3	
○	100	Pudding (NS)	8 oz.
○	80	BlueBerries	2 Cups
	180	**Snack 2 Total**	

2508 — TODAY'S Calorie TOTAL

'NO Sugar & Starch Diet Victory' EZPLAN™   2600 Calories

Day 1 — 2600

DATE:

Record YOUR MORNING Weight:

✓	C:	ITEM:	SERVING:
BREAKFAST			
○	228	POACHED EGGS	3 Large
○	300	Lean P. CHOPS (2)	6 oz.
○	163	Applesauce	14 oz.
○	50	V8 Juice	8 oz.
○	60	Grapefruit	1/2
	801	**Breakfast Total**	
Snack 1			
○	150	Cottage Cheese	10 TBSP
○	80	BlueBerries	2 Cups
	230	**Snack 1 Total**	
Lunch			
○	170	CHICKEN BRST (2)	7.5 oz.
○	50	Grn. SALAD/Drsg	2 Cups
○	110	Blackberries	2 Cups
○	150	Apples Sliced	2 med
	480	**Lunch Total**	
Snack 2			
○	100	Pudding (NS)	8 oz.
○	136	Strawberries (NS)	2 Cups
	236	**Snack 2 Total**	
Dinner			
○	370	Round STEAK (2)	7.5 oz.
○	50	Spin. SALAD/Drsg	2 Cups
○	162	SBerries/BlueB	3 Cups
○	140	Apple Sauce (NS)	12 oz.
	722	**Dinner Total**	
Snack 3			
○	100	Pudding (NS)	8 oz.
○	30	BlueBerries	3/4 Cup
	130	**Snack 3 Total**	

2599 TODAY'S Calorie TOTAL

Day 2 — 2600

DATE:

Record YOUR MORNING Weight:

✓	C:	ITEM:	SERVING:
BREAKFAST			
○	228	POACHED EGGS	3 Large
○	400	Chicken Sausages	4
○	140	Applesauce	12 oz.
○	20	Tomato Juice	4 oz.
○	120	Grapefruit	1 Med
	908	**Breakfast Total**	
Snack 1			
○	100	Pudding (NS)	4 oz.
○	110	Blackberries	2 Cups
	210	**Snack 1 Total**	
Lunch			
○	370	Round STEAK (2)	7.5 oz.
○	50	Spin. SALAD/Drsg	2 Cups
○	108	SBerries/BlueB	2 Cups
○	150	Apples Sliced	2 med
	678	**Lunch Total**	
Snack 2			
○	135	Cottage Cheese	9 TBSP
○	68	Strawberries (NS)	1 Cup
	203	**Snack 2 Total**	
Dinner			
○	255	CHICKEN BRST (3)	11.25 oz.
○	50	Grn. SALAD/Drsg	2 Cups
○	26	Blackberries	1/2 Cup
○	150	Apples Sliced	2 med
	481	**Dinner Total**	
Snack 3			
○	100	Pudding (NS)	8 oz.
○	20	Blueberries (NS)	1/2 Cup
	120	**Snack 2 Total**	

2600 TODAY'S Calorie TOTAL

Day 3 — 2600

DATE:

Record YOUR MORNING Weight:

✓	C:	ITEM:	SERVING:
BREAKFAST			
○	152	POACHED EGGS	2 Large
○	370	Round Steak	7.5 oz.
○	163	Applesauce	14 oz.
○	50	V8 Juice	8 oz.
○	162	SBerries/BlueB	3 Cups
	897	**Breakfast Total**	
Snack 1			
○	100	Raspberries	2 Cup
○	100	Pudding (NS)	8 oz.
	200	**Snack 1 Total**	
Lunch			
○	255	CHICKEN BRST (3)	11.25 oz.
○	50	Grn. SALAD/Drsg	2 Cups
○	100	Asparagus	2 Cups
○	136	Strawberries (NS)	2 Cup
	541	**Lunch Total**	
Snack 2			
○	150	Cottage Cheese	10 TBSP
○	110	Blackberries (NS)	2 Cups
	260	**Snack 2 Total**	
Dinner			
○	300	Lean P. CHOPS	7.5 oz.
○	50	Grn. SALAD/Drsg	1.5 Cups
○	140	Applesauce (NS)	12 oz.
○	76	Peaches Sliced	2 med
	566	**Dinner Total**	
Snack 3			
○	100	Pudding (NS)	8 oz.
○	40	BlueBerries	1 Cup
	140	**Snack 2 Total**	

2604 TODAY'S Calorie TOTAL

'NO Sugar & Starch Diet Victory' EZPLAN™   2600 Calories

Day 4

DATE:

2600 / 4

Record YOUR MORNING Weight:

✓	C:	ITEM:	SERVING:
BREAKFAST			
○	220	EGG Substitute	3 Cups
○	300	Lean P. CHOP (2)	6 oz.
○	163	Applesauce	14 oz.
○	50	V8 Juice	8 oz.
○	120	Grapefruit	1 Med
	853	**Breakfast Total**	
Snack 1			
○	135	Cottage Cheese	9 TBSP
○	80	BlueBerries	1 Cup
	215	**Snack 1 Total**	
Lunch			
○	255	CHICKEN BRST(3)	11.25 oz.
○	50	Grn. SALAD/Drsg.	2 Cups
○	76	Green Beans	2 Cups
○	150	Apple Sliced	2 med
	531	**Lunch Total**	
Snack 2			
○	100	Pudding (NS)	8 oz.
○	136	Strawberries (NS)	2 Cup
	236	**Snack 2 Total**	
Dinner			
○	370	Round STEAK	6.5 oz.
○	50	Spin. SALAD/Drsg.	2 Cups
○	88	Broccoli	2 Cups
○	140	Apple Sauce (NS)	12 oz.
	648	**Dinner Total**	
Snack 3			
○	100	Pudding (NS)	8 oz.
○	20	BlueBerries	1/2 Cup
	120	**Snack 3 Total**	

2603 TODAY'S Calorie TOTAL

Day 5

DATE:

2600 / 5

Record YOUR MORNING Weight:

✓	C:	ITEM:	SERVING:
BREAKFAST			
○	228	POACHED EGGS	3 Large
○	400	Chicken Sausage	4
○	163	Applesauce	14 oz.
○	40	Tomato Juice	8 oz.
○	120	Grapefruit	1 Med
	951	**Breakfast Total**	
Snack 1			
○	100	Pudding (NS)	8 oz.
○	80	BlueBerries	2 Cups
	180	**Snack 1 Total**	
Lunch			
○	255	Chicken BRST (3)	11.25 oz.
○	50	Spin. SALAD/Drsg.	2 Cups
○	108	SBerries/BlueB	2 Cups
○	150	Apples Sliced	2 med
	563	**Lunch Total**	
Snack 2			
○	120	Cottage Cheese	8 TBSP
○	108	SBerries/BlueB	2 Cups
	228	**Snack 2 Total**	
Dinner			
○	300	Lean P. CHOP (2)	6 oz.
○	40	Grn. SALAD/Drsg.	1.5 Cups
○	57	Green Beans	1 1/2 Cups
○	150	Apples Sliced	2 med
	547	**Dinner Total**	
Snack 3			
○	100	Pudding (NS)	7.5 oz.
○	28	Blackberries (NS)	1/2 Cup
	128	**Snack 2 Total**	

2597 TODAY'S Calorie TOTAL

Day 6

DATE:

2600 / 6

Record YOUR MORNING Weight:

✓	C:	ITEM:	SERVING:
BREAKFAST			
○	228	POACHED EGGS	3 Large
○	400	Chicken Sausages	4
○	163	Applesauce	14 oz.
○	50	V8 Juice	8 oz.
○	68	Strawberries	1 Cup
	909	**Breakfast Total**	
Snack 1			
○	100	Raspberries	2 Cup
○	100	Pudding (NS)	8 oz.
	200	**Snack 1 Total**	
Lunch			
○	370	Round STEAK (2)	7.5 oz.
○	50	Grn. SALAD/Drsg.	2 Cups
○	80	Blueberries	2 Cups
○	102	Strawberries (NS)	1 1/2 Cups
	602	**Lunch Total**	
Snack 2			
○	135	Cottage Cheese	9 TBSP
○	110	Blackberries (NS)	2 Cups
	245	**Snack 2 Total**	
Dinner			
○	255	Chicken BRST (3)	11.25 oz.
○	50	Grn. SALAD/Drsg.	2 Cups
○	80	Mom's DRESSING	2 Cups
○	76	Peaches Sliced	2 med
	461	**Dinner Total**	
Snack 3			
○	100	Pudding (NS)	8 oz.
○	80	BlueBerries	2 Cups
	180	**Snack 2 Total**	

2597 TODAY'S Calorie TOTAL

'NO Sugar & Starch Diet Victory' EZPLAN™

Calorie Target

DATE: **DATE:**   **DATE:**

Record YOUR MORNING Weight: Record YOUR MORNING Weight: Record YOUR MORNING Weight:

C: ITEM: SERVING: C: ITEM: SERVING: C: ITEM: SERVING:

BREAKFAST   **BREAKFAST**   **BREAKFAST**

Breakfast Total   Breakfast Total   Breakfast Total

Snack 1   **Snack 1**   **Snack 1**

Snack 1 Total   Snack 1 Total   Snack 1 Total

Lunch   **Lunch**   **Lunch**

Lunch Total   Lunch Total   Lunch Total

Snack 2   **Snack 2**   **Snack 2**

Snack 2 Total   Snack 2 Total   Snack 2 Total

Dinner   **Dinner**   **Dinner**

Dinner Total   Dinner Total   Dinner Total

Snack 3   **Snack 3**   **Snack 3**

Snack 3 Total   Snack 3 Total   Snack 3 Total

TODAY'S Calorie TOTAL   **TODAY'S Calorie TOTAL**   **TODAY'S Calorie TOTAL**

 ISBN 978-0-9800641-8-6

'NO Sugar & Starch Diet Victory' EZPLAN™

Calorie Target

DATE:

Record YOUR MORNING Weight:

✓ C: ITEM: SERVING:

BREAKFAST

○ ___ ___ ___
○ ___ ___ ___
○ ___ ___ ___
○ ___ ___ ___
○ ___ ___ ___

___ Breakfast Total

Snack 1

○ ___ ___ ___
○ ___ ___ ___

___ Snack 1 Total

Lunch

○ ___ ___ ___
○ ___ ___ ___
○ ___ ___ ___
○ ___ ___ ___

___ Lunch Total

Snack 2

○ ___ ___ ___
○ ___ ___ ___

___ Snack 2 Total

Dinner

○ ___ ___ ___
○ ___ ___ ___
○ ___ ___ ___
○ ___ ___ ___

___ Dinner Total

Snack 3

○ ___ ___ ___
○ ___ ___ ___

___ Snack 3 Total

TODAY'S Calorie TOTAL

DATE:

Record YOUR MORNING Weight:

✓ C: ITEM: SERVING:

BREAKFAST

○ ___ ___ ___
○ ___ ___ ___
○ ___ ___ ___
○ ___ ___ ___
○ ___ ___ ___

___ Breakfast Total

Snack 1

○ ___ ___ ___
○ ___ ___ ___

___ Snack 1 Total

Lunch

○ ___ ___ ___
○ ___ ___ ___
○ ___ ___ ___
○ ___ ___ ___

___ Lunch Total

Snack 2

○ ___ ___ ___
○ ___ ___ ___

___ Snack 2 Total

Dinner

○ ___ ___ ___
○ ___ ___ ___
○ ___ ___ ___
○ ___ ___ ___

___ Dinner Total

Snack 3

○ ___ ___ ___
○ ___ ___ ___

___ Snack 3 Total

TODAY'S Calorie TOTAL

DATE:

Record YOUR MORNING Weight:

✓ C: ITEM: SERVING:

BREAKFAST

○ ___ ___ ___
○ ___ ___ ___
○ ___ ___ ___
○ ___ ___ ___
○ ___ ___ ___

___ Breakfast Total

Snack 1

○ ___ ___ ___
○ ___ ___ ___

___ Snack 1 Total

Lunch

○ ___ ___ ___
○ ___ ___ ___
○ ___ ___ ___
○ ___ ___ ___

___ Lunch Total

Snack 2

○ ___ ___ ___
○ ___ ___ ___

___ Snack 2 Total

Dinner

○ ___ ___ ___
○ ___ ___ ___
○ ___ ___ ___
○ ___ ___ ___

___ Dinner Total

Snack 3

○ ___ ___ ___
○ ___ ___ ___

___ Snack 3 Total

TODAY'S Calorie TOTAL

© HCG DIET VICTORY
PLANNER.COM

'NO Sugar & Starch Diet Victory' EZPLAN™

Calorie Target

DATE: **DATE:**   **DATE:**

Record YOUR MORNING Weight: **Record YOUR MORNING Weight:**   **Record YOUR MORNING Weight:**

√   C: ITEM: SERVING: √   C: ITEM: SERVING: √   C: ITEM: SERVING:

BREAKFAST	BREAKFAST	BREAKFAST

_____ Breakfast Total   _____ Breakfast Total   _____ Breakfast Total

Snack 1	Snack 1	Snack 1

_____ Snack 1 Total   _____ Snack 1 Total   _____ Snack 1 Total

Lunch	Lunch	Lunch

_____ Lunch Total   _____ Lunch Total   _____ Lunch Total

Snack 2	Snack 2	Snack 2

_____ Snack 2 Total   _____ Snack 2 Total   _____ Snack 2 Total

Dinner	Dinner	Dinner

_____ Dinner Total   _____ Dinner Total   _____ Dinner Total

Snack 3	Snack 3	Snack 3

_____ Snack 3 Total   _____ Snack 3 Total   _____ Snack 3 Total

TODAY'S Calorie TOTAL   **TODAY'S Calorie TOTAL**   **TODAY'S Calorie TOTAL**

 ISBN 978-0-9800641-8-6

'NO Sugar & Starch Diet Victory' EZPLAN™

Calorie Target

DATE:

Record YOUR MORNING Weight:

✓ C: ITEM: SERVING:

BREAKFAST

○ ____ ____________ ________
○ ____ ____________ ________
○ ____ ____________ ________
○ ____ ____________ ________
○ ____ ____________ ________

____ Breakfast Total

Snack 1

○ ____ ____________ ________
○ ____ ____________ ________

____ Snack 1 Total

Lunch

○ ____ ____________ ________
○ ____ ____________ ________
○ ____ ____________ ________
○ ____ ____________ ________

____ Lunch Total

Snack 2

○ ____ ____________ ________
○ ____ ____________ ________

____ Snack 2 Total

Dinner

○ ____ ____________ ________
○ ____ ____________ ________
○ ____ ____________ ________
○ ____ ____________ ________

____ Dinner Total

Snack 3

○ ____ ____________ ________
○ ____ ____________ ________

____ Snack 3 Total

TODAY'S Calorie TOTAL

DATE:

Record YOUR MORNING Weight:

✓ C: ITEM: SERVING:

BREAKFAST

○ ____ ____________ ________
○ ____ ____________ ________
○ ____ ____________ ________
○ ____ ____________ ________
○ ____ ____________ ________

____ Breakfast Total

Snack 1

○ ____ ____________ ________
○ ____ ____________ ________

____ Snack 1 Total

Lunch

○ ____ ____________ ________
○ ____ ____________ ________
○ ____ ____________ ________
○ ____ ____________ ________

____ Lunch Total

Snack 2

○ ____ ____________ ________
○ ____ ____________ ________

____ Snack 2 Total

Dinner

○ ____ ____________ ________
○ ____ ____________ ________
○ ____ ____________ ________
○ ____ ____________ ________

____ Dinner Total

Snack 3

○ ____ ____________ ________
○ ____ ____________ ________

____ Snack 3 Total

TODAY'S Calorie TOTAL

DATE:

Record YOUR MORNING Weight:

✓ C: ITEM: SERVING:

BREAKFAST

○ ____ ____________ ________
○ ____ ____________ ________
○ ____ ____________ ________
○ ____ ____________ ________
○ ____ ____________ ________

____ Breakfast Total

Snack 1

○ ____ ____________ ________
○ ____ ____________ ________

____ Snack 1 Total

Lunch

○ ____ ____________ ________
○ ____ ____________ ________
○ ____ ____________ ________
○ ____ ____________ ________

____ Lunch Total

Snack 2

○ ____ ____________ ________
○ ____ ____________ ________

____ Snack 2 Total

Dinner

○ ____ ____________ ________
○ ____ ____________ ________
○ ____ ____________ ________
○ ____ ____________ ________

____ Dinner Total

Snack 3

○ ____ ____________ ________
○ ____ ____________ ________

____ Snack 3 Total

TODAY'S Calorie TOTAL

'NO Sugar & Starch Diet Victory' EZPLAN™

Calorie Target

DATE: **DATE:**   **DATE:**

Record YOUR MORNING Weight: **Record YOUR MORNING Weight:**   **Record YOUR MORNING Weight:**

☑ C: ITEM: SERVING: ☑ C: ITEM: SERVING: ☑ C: ITEM: SERVING:

BREAKFAST	**BREAKFAST**	**BREAKFAST**

Breakfast Total   Breakfast Total   Breakfast Total

Snack 1	**Snack 1**	**Snack 1**

Snack 1 Total   Snack 1 Total   Snack 1 Total

Lunch	**Lunch**	**Lunch**

Lunch Total   Lunch Total   Lunch Total

Snack 2	**Snack 2**	**Snack 2**

Snack 2 Total   Snack 2 Total   Snack 2 Total

Dinner	**Dinner**	**Dinner**

Dinner Total   Dinner Total   Dinner Total

Snack 3	**Snack 3**	**Snack 3**

Snack 3 Total   Snack 3 Total   Snack 3 Total

TODAY'S Calorie TOTAL   **TODAY'S Calorie TOTAL**   **TODAY'S Calorie TOTAL**

Section Three:

'Returning to Earth.'

"What lies behind us and what lies before us are tiny matters compared to what lies within us."

Ralph Waldo Emerson

Defeat OBESITY...Forever!

The HCG Assisted 500 Calorie Weight Loss Cure

Section Three: **Introduction: Returning to 'Earth'**

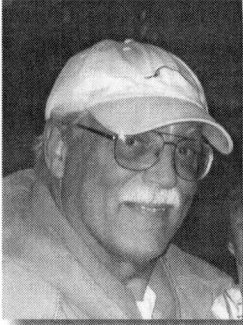

"For four years I did everything the doctor ordered and also began to suffer from a number of different side effects..."

After three years of looking and asking, finally with the help of an enlightened doctor, I found Dr. Simeons..."

"If you are reading these words, it is my hope that you too have defeated obesity..."

Another Drummer?

I love this 'Section Three' quote by Ralph W. Emerson. He is also the one who wrote about **'marching to a different drummer'** which in my mind, is a very appropriate thought when faced with the state of **'modern medicine.'**

Here Is Why I Think We Need Another Option.

My newest grandchild, born in May 2008, is a little girl, and her name is Emerson. When pondering health issues I can't help but think **how close I came** to **never meeting** her, or my next youngest grandchild, Benjamin.

In 2001, what started out as a fun 'sailing school' adventure with my son, quite unexpectedly became **a turning point** in my life. An extensive physical examination was required to join the sailing school. I passed, but with the discovery, that I had become a Type 2 **diabetic**! At that point I began to follow the **'doctors orders'** and went home from my **'big box' doctors** office, with a fistful of prescriptions.

For four years I did **everything** the doctor ordered and also began to suffer from a number of different **side effects** as a result of all of the pills I was popping. **Not fun.**

The **bottom line** is, even after my best efforts, I wound up in **critical condition** laying in a hospital bed, surrounded by specialists, discussing with them the prospect of an induced **coma** and being placed on **life support!** Wow. As I lay pondering their request, the events of recent years, flashed through my mind.

How had I ended up in this predicament? I **resolved** right then and there, that if I survived, I would find **a better solution** for my health quandry. I needed answers.

I came back from the brink and I began to **look**, as they say... **'outside the box.'**

Enter Dr. Simeons' and his 'Weight Loss Cure.'

After about **three years** of looking and asking, finally with the help of an enlightened doctor, I found **Dr. Simeons'** near miraculous, weight loss diet, or as he called it... 'a new approach to obesity.' Wow again.

Only about **a week** into the program I was shocked. I had lost over **20 pounds** and had lowered my blood sugar by over 130 points. I knew then, and I know today, that Dr. Simeons HCG diet protocol was **the 'real deal!'** I have been sharing, the 'HCG answer,' since that moment, and have seen many others come **back** from the **despair of obesity.** When you see that happening, it does get **exciting.**

Victory Over Obesity is Within You.

If you are reading these words, it is my hope that **you** too have **defeated obesity** and are excited about the **new prospects** for your life. Perhaps you will now be around to meet and experience your new little 'bundles of joy' just like I did with my little Emerson and Benjamin, who I **almost missed** the opportunity to meet!

You are on the right track! According to a new 8 year study, **losing just 15 pounds** can cut high blood pressure risks, up to 29% without any medication.

My deepest **congratulations** and **welcome** to the 'HCG alumni club,' where we are all proud to be called 'losers!'

Section Three: **Returning to Earth**

"The 'old doc' is strangely silent on the subject..."

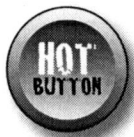

HOT BUTTON

The Silent Dr. Simeons.

The 'old doc' is strangely silent on the subject of **'returning to normal,'** or as I like to call it, **'returning to earth.'** He does refer to a three week **slow re-introduction** of **'sugars'** and **'starches'** but that's about it. A **frighteningly simple release** don't you think? Does that make you wonder... where to go from here?

We're All Illiterate... on Different Subjects.

I found a few things puzzling. The post 'weight setting' **lack of information,** from the old doctor, I just mentioned, is the first one.

Another puzzle is the **unique food selections,** represented by the carefully noted 'four food groups.' Also the **prohibition of 'sugars and starches'** to set our final weight. Not so much the requirements, because I knew they worked... but why?

These things are all a product of **meticulous, trial and error** testing and selection **over 40 years,** and as I have already stated, in my mind are **trustworthy.**

Based on the questions I am getting since the publication of my first book, the **'HCG Victory Tool Kit,'** nearly everyone who completes Dr. Simeons weight loss protocol, wants to know exactly **how** to go on. And wants to find their 'normal.'

"Where do we go from here?"

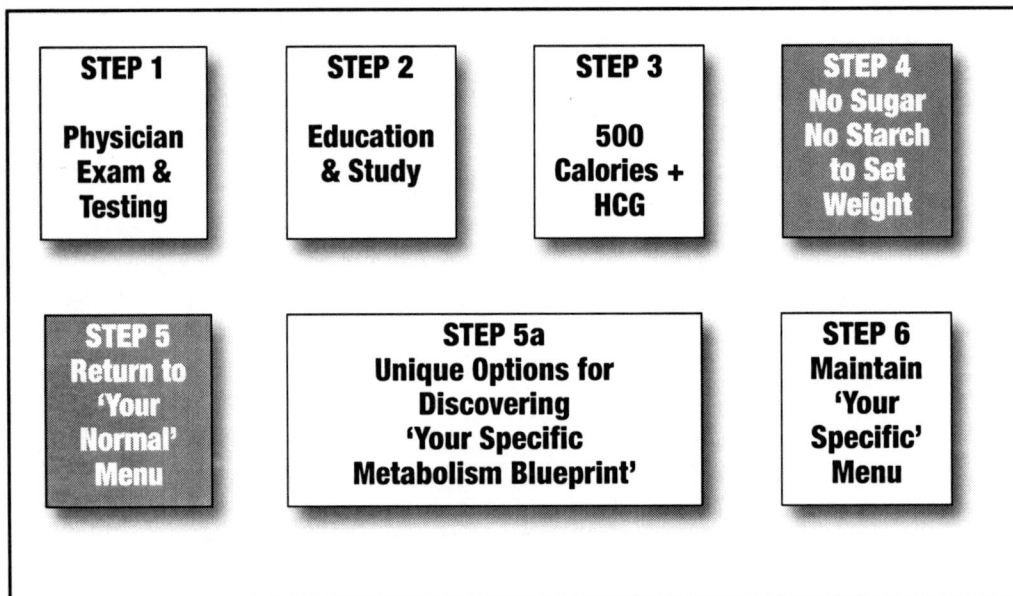

"What is Normal and How Do I Get there?"

STEP 1 Physician Exam & Testing	STEP 2 Education & Study	STEP 3 500 Calories + HCG	STEP 4 No Sugar No Starch to Set Weight

STEP 5 Return to 'Your Normal' Menu	STEP 5a Unique Options for Discovering 'Your Specific Metabolism Blueprint'		STEP 6 Maintain 'Your Specific' Menu

Reviewing The Plan So Far.

Checking your progress chart above, you can see the steps ahead. You should be finishing up with **'Step 4'** and moving to **'Step 5: Return to Your Normal Menu'**

What is "Normal' and How Do I Get There?

HOT BUTTON

First we need to define and layout Dr. Simeons 'return to normal' process and then take a look at what I feel **is the key** to discovering what is **'normal'** for you and for me. It may be different. In fact, I am convinced it will be, if we follow the facts.

I will share the results of my research, for ideas and answers to the questions raised above, as we take a closer look at the **unique nature** of **'metabolism.'**

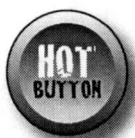

**STEP 5
Return to
'Your
Normal'
Menu**

*"...very slowly
add sugars &
starches always
monitored by
morning
weighing."*

Three Weeks for the Doctor.

We will dig into the question of 'normal' later, but for now, let's stay with **Dr. Simeons definition**. That would be a **minimum 3 week** very slow transition from the 'no sugar or starch' plan to **an unrestricted diet**.

Go Slow & Easy.

The old doctor's advice is pretty brief, he says to, "...very **slowly** add sugars and starches always monitored by morning weighing..."

After finishing 'Step 4' you should know the drill pretty well. It is **a good idea** to either follow your 'no sugar or starch' EZPlans™ or use one of the blank forms, shown at right, **to monitor** your food consumption. Keeping good records is key.

Table 10: Custom Plan Form

Be Deliberate & Calculating.

The best advice I can give you is to **be deliberate** and **plan and record** both your 'unrestricted' sugar or starch intake, and your reactions to it. No question in my mind, that we all react a little differently to foods. This I believe, is because, as I will explain in detail in the pages that follow, we are all **unique** in our **exact** metabolism.

*"The best advice
I can give
you is to be
deliberate & plan
& record..."*

Corrective Action. Live & Learn.

Don't be afraid to use the **'steak day'** or even the **'apple day'** during this transition. Take your time, and stay in your comfort zone. Consulting with your doctor helps.

Your New Found Skill Set.

Let's take a look at the **skills** and **knowledge** you have **mastered**, and important **breakthroughs** you have achieved, while under the influence of the HCG protocol.

- **Better Understanding Of Obesity & The Three Types of Body Fat.**
- **How To Harness Your Body's Natural Weight Control System.**
- **Developing Self Discipline And Control Over What You Eat.**
- **Training in Portion Control & Healthy Food Choices.**
- **How to Defeat Your Personal Obesity & Improve Your Heath Outlook.**
- **How to Kick the Sugar Habit for Good and Why.**
- **How to Plan Your Meals in Both Content & Frequency**
- **Your Correct Daily Caloric Needs & Why.**
- **How to Manage Your Weight & Daily Menus**

*"...a new
adventure into
the world of
metabolism."*

You could probably add to the list. You are now **at a crossroads** in your life. Seize this opportunity and **build** on all of the breakthroughs you have experienced.

Moving Beyond 'Normal.'

Now turn the page for **a new adventure** into the world of **metabolism**. Learn it's **unique nature** and what that may mean for you and me. Let's take a look.

Section Three:	**Finding Your Unique Metabolism**

STEP 5a

A Unique 'Metabolism Blueprint'

"...Does it make sense that what is good for the individual cell is good for the whole body..."

" ...a custom metabolic blueprint..."

"...you or I can be identified as a unique individual out of billions of human beings on the earth."

Understanding Metabolism: The Key to Vigorous Life.

The **process of metabolism** happens when we take on fuel in the form of proteins, carbohydrates & fats and then combining those **food sources** with oxygen, we **'oxidize'** or break them down into their **essential molecular structure**.

Our cells then use these **micro-nutrients** in the form of **vitamins, peptides, sugar, starch, triglycerides and fatty acids,** to grow, build, repair damage, and prosper.

That's life on the celluar level. Our bodies are composed of **untold milllions** of such **tiny 'life units.'** Put them all together and presto, you have a you, or a me.

Okay. Does it make sense that what is **good** for the **individual cell** is good for the **whole body** built of them? Seems logical and reasonable to me. Hold that thought.

Nutritional Element	PROTEINS	CARBS	FATS
Metabolic Impact	The Essential Element of Cell Structure & Power	Primary Source of Energy & Structural Component of Cell Walls & Plasma	Functions as a Structural, Insulating & Energy Storage Component
Structure on the Metabolic Level	Ultimate Source of Peptides & Amino Acids	Ultimately Breaks Down into Sugars & Starches	Ultimately Breaks Down into Triglycerides & Fatty Acids
Common Food Sources	Found in Meats, Poultry & Dairy Foods	Found in Fruits, Grains & Veggies	Found in Cheese, Meats, Nuts & Oils

Table 11: 'Understanding The Basic Elements of Metabolism'

Every Hair on Your Head is Numbered.

Let's take that a step further. What if each of us is made up of a unique combination of **unique cells** in a **unique pattern**. Don't think that's possible? Look at DNA tests.

Using DNA tests you or I can be identified as **a unique individual** out of the billions of human beings on this earth. The hairs on your head **really are** numbered.

I recently, read a report, that our 'tongue prints' are completely unique. (Somebody has way too much time on their hands!) Speaking of hands, fingerprints are another example of our **genetic uniqueness**. Another is the retina in the back of the eye.

More than Skin Deep.

So it isn't a huge stretch to think we are unique **'inside' AND 'out'** all the way down to our individual cells. It follows then, that we each may have a kind of a **'custom metabolic blueprint'** with the abilty to survive and thrive on different diets.

Think of it as different fuel mixtures. Ever notice at the filling station that there are different fuel formulas to choose? Why? To match the fuel needs of the engines.

Our bodies also have unique fuel needs, so we need the correct fuel mixture.

Section Three: **Finding Your Unique Metabolism**

Back to the Future.

It may help to **look at the unique evolution** of 'metabolic medicine.' I believe this will lead us to **some answers** about the significance of 'metabolic profiles.'

Looking into the history of it's evolution is interesting both from the **ground breaking significance** of the entire **metabolic approach** to health, but also the very interesting **parallels and overlaps** with Dr. Simeons **obesity** work.

Dr. Weston Price: The 'Granddaddy of Metabolic Health'

Dr. Weston Price could probably be called the **'grandfather'** of the metabolic approach to better health. He was **a contemporary** of Dr. Simeons and did much of his groundbreaking work at about the same time as the good doctor.

Formally trained as a dentist, Dr. Price became interested in malnutrition and it's impact on health, as he grappled with, what to him was **a contradiciton.** Many of his patients in his Ohio dental practice, **struggled** with tooth decay, gum disease and other odd dental abnormalities, he was aware that people in primitive regions around the world, had **no such 'natural' problems.** He was **curious** as to why that was so, and so in **1934** he began researching the possible causes.

Over and over, Dr. Price discovered, that the indigenous populations he studied had **none of the chronic dieases** that were common place in America. He also made note of the fact, that when these people left their native culture or adapted to **'advanced' diets,** they began **degenerating,** and quickly began developing the same health problems, common in those, theoretically more advanced cultures.

In **1938** he published his findings in a benchmark book entitled, **'Nutrition & Physical Degeneration.'** this was at the same time (1931-1949) that **Dr. Simeons** was working with the poor of India. Not a big stretch of the imagination to think that, living and working in a country full of **malnourished** and **health challenged** people, Dr. Simeons was likely aware of the results of Dr. Price's research.

Dr. Roger Williams: The Dawn of 'Metabolic Profiling'

Another contemporary of Simeons and Price, was **Dr. Roger Williams,** the brilliant biochemist and **discoverer** of vitamin B-5. He contributed a great deal to the emerging **'science of nutrition,'** when he published in **1956,** a book now considered a classic, entitled **'Biochemical Individuality.'**

The **brilliant Dr. Williams** outlined a number of **bold conclusions** as follows:

- Individuality pervades every part of the human body.
- Human beings are highly distinctive in the functioning of their organs and in the composition of their body fluids on every anatomical level.
- Inherited differences extend to the structure and metabolism of every cell and determine the speed and efficiency of their essential functions.
- Unbalanced or inadequate nutrition at the celluar level is a major cause of disease.
- People have genetically determined and highly individualized nutritional requirements.

The insightful doctor, did a very **remarkable** and **shocking** thing. He called for the development of **'metabolic profiles'** which could be used, as a first step, to more effectively evaluate and treat patients utilizing **nutritional ajustments** on a **highly individualized** basis. A **revolutionary** conclusion and dramatic recommendation, by a true **visionary,** writing over 50 years ago.

"Dr. Price could probably be called the 'grandfather' of the metabolic approach..."

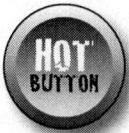

"Another contemporary of Simeons & Price was Dr. Williams."

"...called for the development of 'metabolic profiles' which could be used to evaluate and treat patients..."

Section Three: **Finding Your Unique Metabolism**

"The world of 'mainstream' medicine..."

Yawn of a New Age.

Unfortunately the world of **'mainsteam' medicine** in the decades of the 1940's and 50's was **focusing on the lucrative**, more profitable and rapidly emerging field of **'pharmaceutical science.'** A sad 'fork' in the road scenario, that **has come home** to roost in our present age of **pill popping** and **vaccine crazed** 'modern' medicine.

And so, in spite of **Dr. Williams acknowledged brilliance** and classic contributions as a biochemist, the medical establishment looked at his work and **yawned.**

But, at least **one clinician** out there, was paying attention. It was to be a critical link.

Dr. William D. Kelley: Brilliant Birds of a Feather.

"... a sad 'fork' in the road..."

William D. Kelley held advanced degrees in **biology, chemistry & biochemistry** and graduated from dental college in 1957. He was very much **like** the eminent nutritional pioneer who had gone before him, **Dr. Weston Price,** and was **familar with his work.** The influence of Dr. William's book on Kelley was **significant** in a number of ways. You could say it was for him, **a life changing experience.**

Kelley was **a gifted researcher, clinician** and **brilliant innovator.** He also had a good grasp of Dr. Price's theories, as he began his own research. As Price had done before him, he began **questioning** the **root causes** behind the **many dental abnormalities** he encountered in his practice.

Little did he realize the **impact** the work of **Dr. Price** and **Dr. Williams** would have for him **personally.** In fact, as a biochemist, it was to be his **'acid test.'**

Willian D. Kelley held advanced degrees in biology, chemistry & biochemistry..."

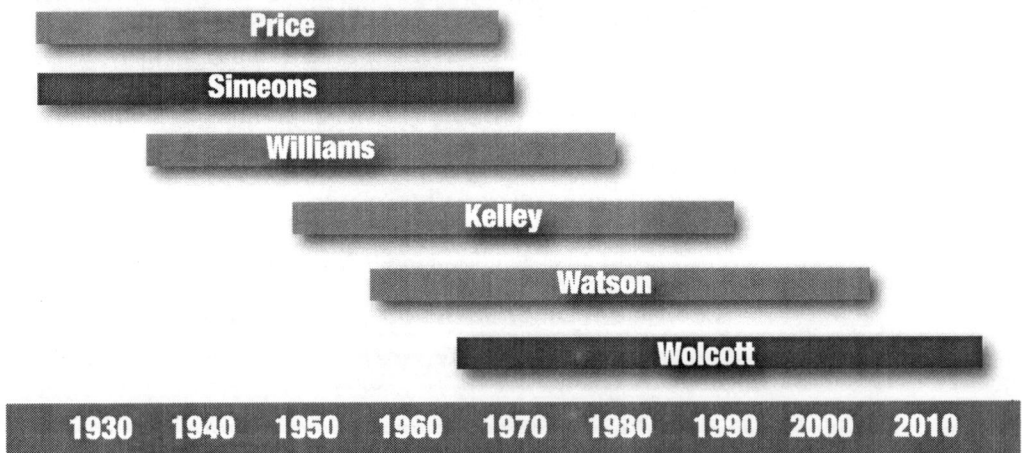

Smart Doctors on Parade: 'Thinking Outside the Box'

Price
Simeons
Williams
Kelley
Watson
Wolcott

| 1930 | 1940 | 1950 | 1960 | 1970 | 1980 | 1990 | 2000 | 2010 |

Table 12: 'Marching to the Tune of A Different Drummer.'

The above illustration charts the approximate working lives of the brilliant doctors, dentists, scientists and pioneers who have advanced the science of 'metabolic profile studies' over the last 80 plus years. Also shown is the parallel working lifetime of Dr. A.T.W. Simeons the discoverer of the HCG assisted weight loss protocol and other significant contributions to humanity, in the areas of research and treatment, for malaria, bubonic plaque and leprosy.

Section Three: **Finding Your Unique Metabolism**

The Acid Test: Mother Knows Best.

Dr. Kelley was not quite 40 years old, when he went home from his own personal physicians office, with **grim news** for his family. He had been diagnosed with the most aggressive form of pancreatic cancer. This was in the mid 1960's and was considered untreatable. Thus, he was given **mere months to live**.

"He had been diagnosed with the most aggressive form of pancreatic cancer."

One member of Kelley's family took charge in the crisis and **refused to accept** the prognosis. His mother was a no nonsense lady, who had grown up on a farm during tough times. She was poorly educated, but full of common sense, and had little use for doctors. Using her **natural smarts** and good sense she demanded that her son, who had very poor eating habits, abandon the **junk food** and revert to an exclusive diet of **carbohydrates**, consisting of fresh fruits, veggies and whole grains.

Kelley followed his mother's plan, and much to his surprise, he began to feel better, had more energy and **his tumors began to shrink**. Encouraged by his success he began research into the impact of whole, natural, non-toxic foods and nutritional treatments for cancer. Over the years ahead he used himself as a guinea pig.

Eight years later **he cured his wife** of the after effects of toxic paint exposure, but this time, it was a **protein heavy diet** of meat and meat broths. In fact, he observed as he tried to cure her using carbohydrates, she had worsened.

Eureka: 'Unique Metabolism Types.'

"...a diet that was good and healthy for some had the opposite effect on others."

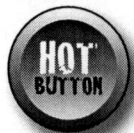

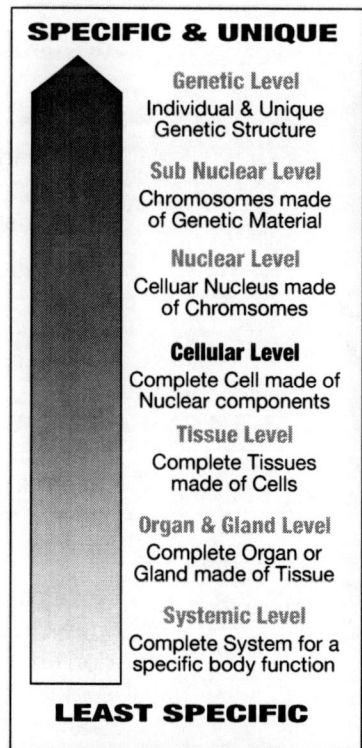

Dr. Kelley had passed the acid test and made a great discovery. It was crystal clear to him that a diet that was good and **healthy for some** had the opposite effect on others. Following that concept to it's logical conclusion, he invented exactly what **Dr. Williams** had prescribed back in the 1950's, **a clinical tool** for assessing the **unique metabolisms** of individuals.

Due to his ground breaking work, he is regarded as the **'father of metabolic typing.'**

Remember the Gas Pump Illustration?

What Dr. Kelley had **discovered & confirmed** in a very dramatic way, was the need for different or **unique fuels,** for different or **unique human engines.** In fact, the individual cell, is the little 'engine of life,' in the hierarchy of the human body.

Why is this Important?

This is important to us as we determine our unique **metabolism** and place our trust in it to determine what our **'metabolic blueprint'** is and what types of foods will lead us to **optimum health & weight** management, as you shall see on the next few pages. A **healthy properly fueled cell** is the goal.

SPECIFIC & UNIQUE

Genetic Level
Individual & Unique
Genetic Structure

Sub Nuclear Level
Chromosomes made
of Genetic Material

Nuclear Level
Celluar Nucleus made
of Chromsomes

Cellular Level
Complete Cell made of
Nuclear components

Tissue Level
Complete Tissues
made of Cells

Organ & Gland Level
Complete Organ or
Gland made of Tissue

Systemic Level
Complete System for a
specific body function

LEAST SPECIFIC

**Table 13: Hierarchy of
The Human Body**

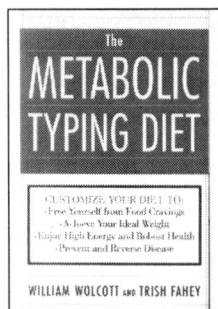

"To be honest, I had no idea I could feel as good as I started to feel..."

"...he could eat no fat... his wife could eat no lean..."

"...recall from Dr. Simeons protocol the 'ANS' controls all of those body functions..."

William Wolcott: Critical Parts of the Puzzle.

Wolcott went to work for Dr. Kelley after hearing his presentation in 1977. He saw first hand, both **personally** and **professionally** the truth and effectiveness of Kelley's metabolic protocol. Amazed at the effectiveness of the treatment, he wrote, "To be honest, I had no idea I could feel as good as I started to feel..." Since that time, over the intervening years, he has dedicated his life to furthering the science of **'metabolic typing.'**

Reviewers now describe William Wolcott as the **world's leading authority** on metabolic typing and the central figure advancing that area of dietary science.

In his excellent book, **'The Metabolic Typing Diet'** written with Trish Fahey, he shares how he studied the works of Dr. Kelley and tried to reconcile the methods and successes of his practice, with the work of a clinical psychologist named, Dr. George Watson, who was also very successful, in treating mental conditions, using a nutritional approach.

Another New Solution 'Outside the Box.'

Wolcott's dilemna was the fact that **both systems worked** but seemed to be in conflict with each other. After exhaustive studies he concluded that both men were right and part of **a third solution**. Another piece had been added to the puzzle.

Breaking Down Wolcott's Dilemna.

A basic understanding of the solutions developed by Kelley and Watson, and their integration by William Wolcott, into a multi-dimensional **metabolic solution**, is necessary, to fully understand the impact for you and me in our search for **'normal.'**

The 'Fork' in the Road.

Remember the experience of Dr. Kelley and his wife? In a variation of the nursery rhyme... **'he could eat no fat, his wife could eat no lean...'** their fuel needs were 180 degrees apart. Now that must have made dinner time at the Kelley's a very interesting experience, but what we need to look at is, where did he go from there?

Kelley was at a 'fork' in the road, in the dietary sense of the word, but didn't know it. He continued to pursue the metabolic solution, especially a way to quantfy or predetermine a persons correct metabolic type, and from that identify the raw materials to seek and avoid, **to achieve optimum health and vitality** on the celluar level, thereby affecting the entire body. A simple, but medically earthshaking, concept.

Kelley turned to the study of the 'autonomic nervous sytem' or 'ANS.' If you recall from **Dr. Simeons protocol**, the 'ANS' controls all of those body functions that you don't have to think about to do. For example such things as breathing, digestion & metabolism. Remember how we used the **HCG + 500 Calorie diet** to affect the brain's **hypothalumus**? That is the is the reason for HCG's effectiveness.

Fascinating to me how all of these **great minds** overlap and parallel each other, all from a different perspective, and all very successfully proven in the arena of human experience. They certainly are **brilliant** birds of a feather. **(See Table 12)**

"...opposing and at the same time complementary forces... just ask Darth Vader."

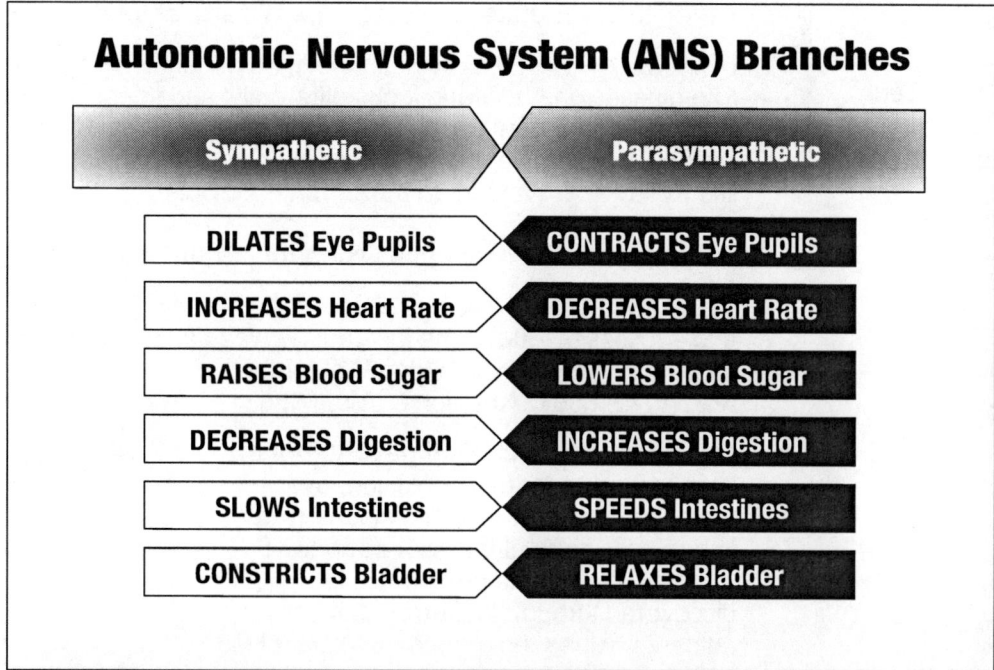

Autonomic Nervous System (ANS) Branches

Sympathetic	Parasympathetic
DILATES Eye Pupils	CONTRACTS Eye Pupils
INCREASES Heart Rate	DECREASES Heart Rate
RAISES Blood Sugar	LOWERS Blood Sugar
DECREASES Digestion	INCREASES Digestion
SLOWS Intestines	SPEEDS Intestines
CONSTRICTS Bladder	RELAXES Bladder

Table 14: Illustration of Sympathetic VERSUS Parasympathetic Functions

The Autonomic System: A Story of Opposing Forces.

Light versus dark. Hot versus cold. Positive versus negative. On versus off. It is easy to see that **opposing and at the same time complementary** forces are everywhere we look. Just ask Darth Vader.

A perfect example of that, is the autonomic nervous system (ANS). As Dr. Simeons and Dr. Kelley understood, the 'ANS' is the '**master regulator of metabolism.**'

Dr. Kelley pursued **the answers** to determining individual metabolic needs, or for our purposes, finding out what **our** 'normal' should be.

"...for our purposes finding out what our normal should be."

He succeeded to a degree, and was the **first researcher** to step around 'additives' such as vitamins and supplements. He began seeking to replace them with the proper '**raw material**' as he put it. Much like Dr. Simeons had concluded that obesity didn't necessarily occur because people over ate, but that they over ate because they were obese, Dr. Kelley believed that the additives only **masked** severe **eating imbalances**. Remember, he almost died from 'poor eating habits.'

He was looking for **a cure not a treatment**. Hurray for Dr. Kelley!

Puzzling though, were **his failures** and the fact that sometimes his approach only made things worse. The stage was set for '**Wolcott the Wizard**'

STEP 6 Maintain 'Your Specific' Menu

Filling in the Blanks: Wolcott, 'The Wizard' of 'Metabolic Typing.'

Have you ever seen a movie in the 'third dimension?' When you put those funny little glasses on, the world looks differently, and things that were fuzzy and out of focus take on **a new form.** That's kind of what William Wolcott did to the world of metabolic typing, he moved it from the single dimension championed by pioneers like Kelley and Watson, to **a multifaceted science**, that is hard to ignore.

Dr. Watson & the 'Personal Oxidation' Solution.

You recall Wolcott's dilemma. He couldn't resolve Dr. George Watson's methods and successes, due to the fact that he was using a **seemingly contradictory** approach. Wolcott discovered Watson by reading his book, 'Nutrition & Your Mind.'

"Wolcott... ...moved it from the single dimension... to a multifaceted science..."

Dr. Watson was **a clinical psychologist,** who had come to the conclusion, over many years of practice, that biochemical imbalances were at the **root causes** of many of his patients problems. He discovered through trial error, that certain nutrients helped the emotional states of his patients, but **the same nutrients** had the **opposite effect** on others.

Unlike Kelley he didn't turn to the 'auto-nomic system' for classifying his patients and determining their needs, instead he choose to examine **'celluar oxidation.'** He had discovered a distinct relationship between peoples **emotional and psychological characteristics** and the rate at which their **cells converted nutrients** to energy.

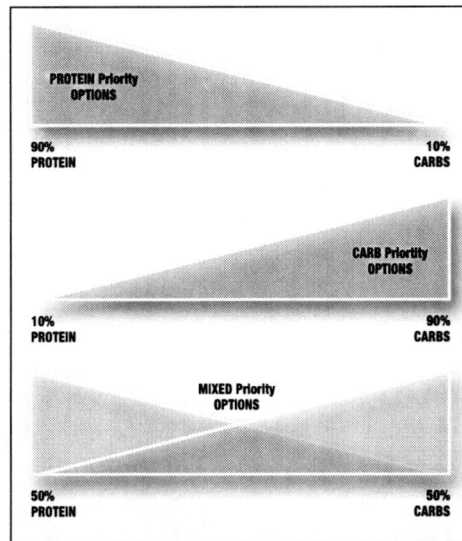

Table 15: Three Oxidation Types

"That is exactly the phenomena, in his search for a solution, that Dr. Watson focused on."

It is ironic, when you recall, **Dr. Kelley**, who thrived on a heavy carbs diet, but his wife, was very protein centered. That is exactly the phenomena, in his search for a solution, that **Dr. Watson** focused on. Both Dr. Kelley's **'autonomic system'** centered approach, and Dr. Watson's **'celluar oxidation,'** represented dimensions of what would be the ultimate answer.

One Plus One Equals Three.

Wolcott **solved the dilemma** and went on to add more **dimensions** and depth to the world of 'metabolic typing.' He realized that there was a balance, or dominance factor, between the **'autonomic system'** and the **'celluar oxidation'** rate.

The 'Dominance Factor.'

Here's how he describes the **'dominance factor,'** " Whether you are 'autonomic dominant' or 'oxidative dominant' will determine **how a food or nutrient behaves** in your body..." After another 10 years of study, he determined seven additional parameters, greatly increasing the **precision and depth** of the technology.

Section Three: **Finding Your Unique Metabolism**

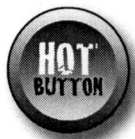

Summary of Conclusions & Options.

Okay. We just covered an **overview of metabolism**. Hopefully you have a working understanding of what it is and what it means to your weight and health as you seek to **return to 'normal.'** I suspect many of us are like William Wolcott, that is we don't have a clue to what it feels like to be healthy and vital, since we are not realizing our health potential. Somewhere along the way **we have lost it** and most likely it is due to the **'raw materials,'** as Dr. Kelley said, that we are supplying to our little 'engines of life,' our cells, which are simply put, **the key to health**.

Taking that to the next step takes us closer to our objective. Our bodies are constructed, maintained and repaired by a colllection of millions of cells. Improve the health of **your cells** and improve your health. Then consider that each one of us is as **unique inside** as we are on the outside, which leads to the logical conclusion that our 'fuel mixture' for **optimum** performance is also very unique, and we are at the threshold of defining what is **'normal'** for each of us.

The final piece of the puzzle needed is a method of predicting with precision exactly what our **metabolic blueprint** is and the types of foods to use and avoid to reach our potential on a celluar level. Then we could experience 'normal' in all of it's glory.

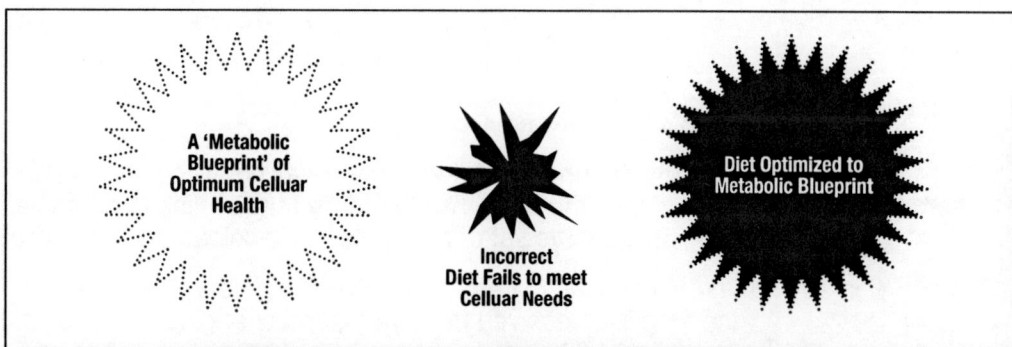

"...we are not realizing our health potential"

"...needed is a method of predicting with precision exactly what our metabolic blueprint is..."

A 'Metabolic Blueprint' of Optimum Celluar Health

Incorrect Diet Fails to meet Celluar Needs

Diet Optimized to Metabolic Blueprint

Table 16: Optimizing The Metabolic Blueprint™

Here's Why I am Sharing These Concepts.

" This metabolic approach to better health is well founded..."

No, I don't own stock in William Wolcott's company, although I probably should. My motivation in sharing all of this is the same as my motivation for sharing more about Dr. Simeons work, **I believe he is right,** and is offering a far better solution than you will ever find in 'mainstream medicine.' It can be life changing.

Discovering the **uniqueness** of your individual metabolic blueprint using Wolcott's metabolic typing system, after completing Dr. Simeons HCG weight loss protocol is a great decision. It answers the question '...where do I go from here.' It opens up a whole **world of possibilities** for you and for me. Uniquely of course.

This **metabolic** approach to better health, which by the way naturally results in **weight control,** was founded and developed by a group of brilliant biochemists, dentists, psychologists, nutritionists and reserachers over the last 80 some years. In Wolcott's book he shares in depth many **case histories** and lays out a detailed and fascinating description of it's development over the last 8 decades. His book is a real heavy weight, as he is probably the top expert in the field today.

Section Three: **Finding Your Unique Metabolism**

"Above are a few of the reports I received after completing the online Metabolic Typing™ survey."

"I can see the common denominators in Dr. Simeons and William Wolcott's protocols..."

Steps to Take in the Right Direction.

If you want to pursue it further here are some optional actions to take.

1) Buy the book by Wolcott & Fahey, 'The Metabolic Typing Diet'

Study the book until you are ready to move on. It is more of a reference work and contains a lot more 'protein' than 'carbs,' if you know what I mean. In the book you will find a much more in depth coverage of the entire procedure and a 'self evaluation' test.

2) Log on to Wolcott's website.

There you will find more information and the opportunity to purchase a deeper evaluation which includes a lot of helpful guides and resources. See **Appendix A** for more information.

a) If you order the profile you can download and follow the very complete instructions provided. Good for the long haul.

b) Be patient, this does not work overnight. You will be offered some optional ways to supplement the process if you choose to.

c) They actually have consultants or advisors around that you can contact. Some of them work for a fee.

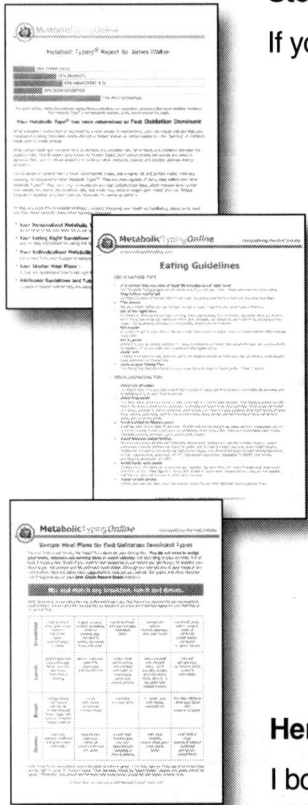

Here's What I Have Done.

I bought the book. Studied it until I was convinced. I then completed the self test contained in the book. Next I ordered the on-line in depth version and received a **very impressive** set of materials, to download and use. Their website explains.

I have changed my **eating habits** and personal menus as a result. I am following the food list I received from them, and changing the ratios of protein, carbs and fats accordingly. Of course, I had changed my eating habits as a direct result of my HCG experience, to a healthier, natural and lower sugar and starch approach, so the change wasn't too drastic. This is why I am presenting this material at this point, because **the timing should be right**, for just about any **HCG alumni**.

I definitely do feel more **alert** and sharper mentally and I do sleep better. On a personal note, I have recently been through a great deal of stress, providing hospice care as my mother passed away at home, and I have been calm through that experience. It is very much of an '**at peace** with everything' feeling, even though I fell behind in the completion of this planner, I didn't get stressed out.

As I understand it, the **metabolic process** takes time to fully mature and will result in achieving **optimum weight control** as well, so based on the experience so far, I am looking forward to that with anticipation as I follow my recommended plan.

Conclusion.

I hope you are considering the **'metabolic blueprint'** options presented here. I believe it is a viable and reasonable next move after finishing the HCG weight loss protocol. I am not a doctor, but I can certainly **see the truth**. I can see the common denominators in Dr. Simeons' and William Wolcott's protocols. They are both right.

Appendix A :

'Helpful References.'

"Refusing to be side-tracked by an all too facile interpretation of obesity, I have always held that overeating is the result of the disorder, not its cause..."

Dr. A.T.W. Simeons

Defeat OBESITY...Forever!

The HCG Assisted 500 Calorie Weight Loss Cure

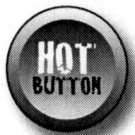

"In my opinion the HCG diet protocol is not a do-it-yourself kit."

"Basically there are seven areas here to look at..."

"They are more interested in treating the symptoms and selling supplements and multiple medications to the chronically obese... than curing them forever."

The 'Worldwide Web,' A Blessing and a... Curse!

The computer revolution is over... they won!

A lot of stuff on the internet is 'junk' and even obscene. However the positive side of the **computer revolution** and the world wide web is the tremendous access to information. Lots and lots of it. Many of you likely discovered **this book** in that way.

The purpose of this section is to help you use the 'web' as an **efficient tool** to support and complement your HCG weight loss adventure. To that end I have weeded out and found some helpful websites for you.

This not an exhaustive list, but it is the essence of what can be helpful for you and I. Remember, **we are after simpler**... not harder.

Basically there are **seven areas** areas here to look at:

(1) Websites: General Food & Nutrition Information

(2) Specific Products and Brands (tested & recommended)

(3) Some 'local organic produce' Locators.

(4) Why You Should Choose 'organic produce'.

(5) Websites: Specific to the 'HCG Weight Loss.'

(6) Websites: Related to Health & Nutritional Education & Evaluation

(7) Bonus. 'HCG Conforming' Basic Recipes & Preparation

A Necessary Word of Caution.

Here's **something that concerns me**. I feel It is a **justified** and **ethical** concern.

On the **web** you will find **all kinds** of HCG offers. Some of them offering to sell you 'direct without a prescription' HCG and a variety of other products. In my opinion the HCG diet protocol is **not a do-it-yourself** kit. It is meant to be **physician** directed.

I don't know who these people are. Some of them are probably sincere and have the best of intentions for you. To others you are just **their prey**. Don't be.

The **HCG + 500C** plan is a legitimate medical breakthrough that should not be sullied by shady operators. There are those in the 'fat industry,' who make their living from touting various 'fad diets,' who would love to ban HCG usage. Don't help their case.

They are more interested in treating the symptoms and selling supplements and multiple medications to the chronically obese... than curing them forever. Beware.

I am not a medical doctor, but I do have enough common sense to know that you are messing with a **critical part of your brain** that controls all of your body processes.

Do you want to **be victorious** and get control of your obesity? Find yourself an **enlightened doctor** directed program. Your **HCG supplies** should come from a **legitimate local pharmacy**.

| Appendix A | Helpful REFERENCES: Food Websites |

Here's **a few food related sites** I find helpful and **a brief summary** of the content.

You **do not need** all of **this information** to be victorious with your **doctor** directed **HCG diet plan**. But for those of you who want the, "...rrrrest of the story," as Paul Harvey used to say, here you go.

General Food Information:

"...reseacrh to your hearts content..."

www.fns.usda.gov/fsn/

Your tax dollars at work. A kind of an umbrella site that allows you to research to your hearts content. Lots of background information and not a lot of 'spin.'

www.oph-good-housekeeping.com/food-nutrition.html

"I like the searchable content by food categories..."

I like the searchable content by food categories, which allows you to look up an item (i.e. 'Fruits' and get a rundown by Calories, fat, carbs, protein and Nutritional value. Also has a good Q and A. section. I rate them fairly neutral.

Organic Foods:

www.eatwild.com

"...grass fed beef, poultry, pork & dairy..."

Information and sources for 'grass fed' beef, poultry, pork and dairy foods. Also for the adventurous... bison! (that would be buffalo to most of us) By the way buffalo is very good for you if you can find it locally. A commercial site.

www.organic-center.org

Pro organic stance and funded by natural food producers. Very knowledge-able site with lots of insight into the value of organic foods and methods.

www.organicvalley.coop/

"...has a very good searchable, stre-house of data and reserach..."

Another commercial site sponsored by organic food producers. Has a very good searchable, storehouse of data and research, on both the reasons to 'eat organic' and 'avoid non-organic' foods. Impressive content.

Local Produce Locators

The organic food issue begs the question... "Where can I get local organic food?"

www.LocavoreNetwork.com

"...find a local source for the type of produce you want, you can contact the farm through this site."

Odd name but a memorable one. This is the only comprehensive nation wide data base for over 15,000 farmers and the public sector. You can not only **find a local source** for the type of produce you want, you can **contact** the farm through this site. New and creating a lot of excitement. Holy cow!

Even includes **proper etiquette** to use when visiting a farm. Started out as one 'produce loving' man's hobby and mushroomed. **Interesting**.

Appendix C   **Helpful REFERENCES: Why Organic?**

This Doesn't Look Like Kansas, ToTo!

Young Dorothy and her little doggie, found themselves whisked away to the land of OZ, where among other things, she learned that all questions would be answered if she just "...followed the **'yellow brick road.'** We all know how that turned out.

The 'Wizard' turned out to be a phony and a fake and the Emerald City... well, it just wasn't what it appeared to be. In the end it was all just one big dream... or was it?

"Now much of our food supply is 'phoney' and 'fake' and isn't good for us.

We have all been following our own 'yellow brick road,' trusting the bureaucrats and the **big food companies** to take care of everything. Now much of our food supply is 'phoney' and 'fake' and isn't good for us. It **looks good** but is **mainly a facade.**

There is No Place Like Home.

Organic growers, farmers and food producers are attempting to get us back home on the farm, away from the nearly **600 pesticides** used in agriculture production. Synthetic chemicals are in everything we eat. More safety concerns appear daily.

Organic farmers believe that the strongest plants and healthiest livestock thrive without the added chemicals. Thus the 'organic' industry avoids these practices.

Just as learning how to eat healthy is important to your body's health, so to, is what kind of food you eat. Garbage in... garbage out. **Eat a chemical... be a chemical.**

"...learning how to eat healthy is important to your body's health."

Somewhere Over the Rainbow.

Have you ever tasted a vine ripened tomato picked at it's peak after being allowed to ripen in it's own time? How about a tree ripened apple or peach? The same concept is true of farm animals who are allowed to grow at their own natural pace without artificial stimulants or hormones. That's what 'organic food' is all about.

As it turns out, there is **a direct connection** between **flavor** and **nutrition.**

Nutrient rich soil, clean water, good feed, healthy pastures. Not surprising is it?

Courage, Brains, and a Heart.

In my opinion you should choose **organic** products for the foods you eat day in and day out. Patronize **your local organic farm** producers. Check out **page 158** of this section for **web sites** to locate organically produced products.

"...you should choose organic products for the foods you eat day in and day out."

If you have any doubts about the **increased nutritional values** in organic foods, check out the facts and figures via the websites referenced in this section.

Having all of the **chemical influences** absorbed into our body from **non-organic** foods no doubt **contributes to** our obesity problem by **altering** our **sensitive natural weight management** system.

If you use your **brain**, you know, **it is smart** to eat **organic.**

In your **heart**, you know it's the right thing to do. Especially for the foods you eat most often. **Be courageous** and do the right thing. Don't fear the 'flying monkeys.'

There really is '...no place like home!'

Appendix A   **Helpful REFERENCES: Food Sources**

Recommended Products & Food Sources

Here is a short list of product brands I have **tested and used** and found to be great quality, tasty and very usable in the various phases of the diet.

"...brands I have tested and used and found to be great quality, tasty and usable in the various phases of the diet."

Table A-1: Tested Food, Produce & Seasonings with Website Address			
www.site	Products for: HCG + 500	NS/NS	Life
www.Annie'sNaturals.com	YES	YES	YES
www.Bragg.com	YES	YES	YES
www.FrontierCoop.com	YES	YES	YES
www.GoodEarth.com	YES	YES	YES
www.OrganicVilleFoods.com	YES	YES	YES
www.TreeTop.com	YES	YES	YES
www.WildOrganics.net	YES	YES	YES
www.WaldenFarms.com	YES	YES	YES
www.HGOFarms.com	YES	YES	YES
www.NaturipeFarms.comt	YES	YES	YES
www.SausagesByAmylu.com	YES	YES	YES
www.ColemanNatural.com	YES	YES	YES
www.OregonsWildHarvest.com	YES	YES	YES
www.North-Wood-Buffalo.com	YES	YES	YES

"Most all of them are organic..."

"...they put their money where their mouth is..."

The list here is just a short one to get you started in the right direction.

Most all of them, not only are organic, but have links to other companies and co-op's that are in the same category. You will find a wide range of foods, seasonings and natural sweetening products that are HCG safe. It's a link to a whole new, safer world.

Some are financially supportive of organic farming and organic co-ops in the USA. So they put their money where their mouth is!

Appendix A   **Helpful REFERENCES: Health & Nutritional**

"You can likely find the answers to your questions..."

Expanding Your Horizons: HCG & Unique Metabolic Typing® Resources.

On this page you can likely find the **answers** to your questions about the HCG protocol or William Wolcott's, metabolic nutritional typing, research and applications.

HCG 'Victory Collection' Books & Guides.

There are a number of books in the **HCG Victory Collection** published by GreatNewsPress.com. If you didn't notice, below is a listing of our websites.

www.HCGVictoryToolKit.com

This is book one in the series and is centered on the basic concepts and provides an easy to follow success track. Emphasis in this guide is how to get off to the **right start** with Dr. Simeons '**prescription** for weight loss.'

www.HCGVictoryPlanner.com

Book two in the series. The major emphasis is streamlining and saving time and staying on course during the **'weight setting'** step in the HCG diet. Features pre-made **EZPlan™** menu plans for a genuine turn-key solution. Goes beyond weight setting and breaks new ground in the area of returning ways to return to **'normal'** with a survey of unique 'metabolic blueprints.'

"Great websites, helpful books & Special Reports"

Great NewsPress.com on line Special Reports.

Accessable through the **'HCG VictoryToolKit.com' website.** You will find a library of **topical papers** on on Dr. Simeons 'HCG Assisted Weight Loss.'

www.OralHCG.com

Dr. Daniel Belluscio is regarded as the world's greatest living expert on the HCG assisted weight loss method. Everything (including pictures) that you were afraid to ask about the proctocol. Very sucessful with oral HCG.

Metabolic Study Resources.

William Wolcott founded 'HealthExcel' an organization that provides technical consulting service to health professionals. Also listed here are his consumer websites for **Metabolic Typing®** services, education and support.

www.healthexcel.com or **www.MetabolicTyping.com**

Wolcott's additional support sites for metabolic education and nutritional supplies.

www.CustomizeYourDiet.com
www.MetabolicEd.com
www.CustomNutritionSystems.com

A site for 'Metabolic Studies' historical archives, a non-profit foundation. Very cool. They publish a monthly newsletter and distribute books and tapes on nutrition.

www.price-pottenger.org

A Brilliant Book!

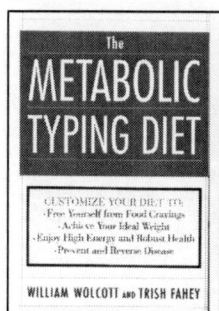

The METABOLIC TYPING DIET
CUSTOMIZE YOUR DIET TO:
- Free Yourself from Food Cravings
- Achieve Your Ideal Weight
- Enjoy High Energy and Robust Health
- Prevent and Reverse Disease

WILLIAM WOLCOTT and TRISH FAHEY

ISBN 978-0-7679-0564-0

Appendix A	REFERENCE: Helpful Recipes & Techniques

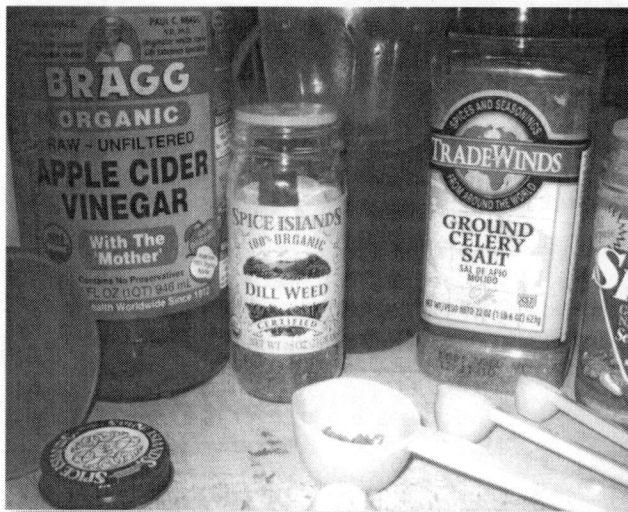

Shown here are some of the things you will need to make your 'Mom in a Bottle' dressing a success.

Taste Tested Tips & Techniques

Fresh fruit will normally be a part of the **basic salad recipes** which adds some **natural sweetness** and flavor.

You can use **any variety of apple** so experiment until you find a few favorites. **Refrigerate apples** as soon as you get them home. Always store at **42-45 degrees** to preserve the quality and crispness of your apples.

'Mom in a Bottle' Apple Cider Vinegar All Purpose Dressing

Summary of this Tested Recipe:

Organic Apple Cider Vinegar dressing is your friend. This all purpose **salad dressing** will be a stalwart in your **tool kit**. Take some time and **perfect it**.

You will come to love it.

Adding your favorite **sugarless seasonings** to personalize it, is part of the fun.

I like the tartness of the **Apple Cider Vinegar,** so I skipped the sweetener. Do some tasting and you will find the right combination for your taste buds.

Keep in mind as you eat the allowed foods and flavorings, **your taste buds will sharpen** and you may want to adjust the formula.

When you are done it will taste just like **mom** made it.

Write down **your ingredients** and put the top on it and put it in the fridge. Always better when chilled.

You can use this dressing on **salads** and on **meats**. It adds very few **calories** and all of the benefits of natural **'organic vinegar.'**

What You Will Need:

Apple Cider Vinegar
Organic Raw & Unfiltered with the 'Mother' in the bottle.

Purified Water
Filtered or bottled

Sugarless Seasonings
Check the ingredients on the label for any hidden sugars. Your preference. See suggestions below.

Mixing Bottle with cap
Used to mix the ingredients and shake and store for use on your salads.

Keep Refrigerated

The Recipe:

4 oz. Apple Cider Vinegar
Organic Raw & Unfiltered with the 'Mother' in it.

8 oz. Pure Water

Seasonings Choices
1/2 tsp Celery Salt
1/4 tsp Onion salt
Dash of Dill Weed
Dash of Garlic Salt

Optional:
Natural sweetener such as Agave Nectar or Liquid Stevia.

Fresh 'Organic' Lemon

Here's What You Do:

Measure and add **water** and **vinegar** to your **mixing bottle**. Start adding the **basic seasonings** in the amounts suggested and then **season to your taste** buds. Be sure to shake well. The dressing will be a little tart by itself. If it is too tart, you may like the **optional sweeteners**. I prefer the Agave, some like Stevia instead. Go slow. These natural sweeteners are **very strong** compared to sugar. A little goes a long way. Fresh **Lemon juice** is optional.

The flavors of the **lettuce** and **apples** and **meat** in the finished salad will modify it. It's best to taste test after application to your salad recipe. Cap it up and chill. There you have it... **'Mom in a Bottle.'** Shake well before **each** use.

2 oz = 10 Calories

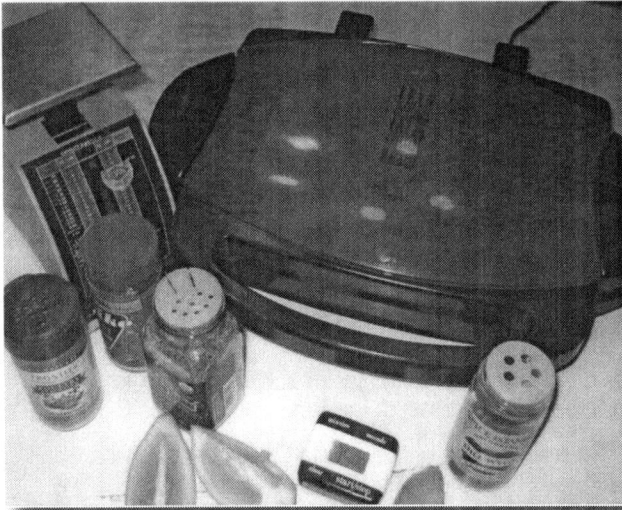

Shown above is my favorite model of the George Foreman Grill. Works very well. I prefer the model with the removable parts. Makes cleaning much simpler and easier.

Getting 'Mean' with Protein.

Summary:

Since you obviously are **trimming and weighing** your meat while **raw,** it follows that some type of cooking is required and there are a few choices to make.

This page **covers the basics** of preparing your **PROTEIN** focusing on 'Preparation' and 'Cooking Methods' Covered are **barbecue, broiling, baking** or using the infamous George Foreman "...lean... mean... grillin'...machine."

We'll look at the pluses and minuses of these methods. Plus some **tips** and **techniques.**

This should help with preparing your chosen source of protein, and achieving the necessary variety and rotation needed for your **HCG + 500 Calorie** menu plan.

Here are some guidelines.

What You Will Need:

Gas Grill barbecue
Cooking in **batches** is recommended. A gas grill is more convenient and pollution free. Much **easier to control** the temperature consistently. A Built in thermometer is a big plus.

Oven or Broiler Oven
Use your oven for baking and broiling. A broiler oven will work as well.

George Foreman Grill
Lots of different models. I like the larger ones with the **removable** cooking plates for ease of cleaning. A good investment.

Your 'Sugar Free' Seasonings
Go on a shopping expedition and stock up on **sugar free seasoning** for meat. You can find them everywhere. Some are labeled **'Poultry or Steak Seasoning'** some are flavored for general use.

Portable Kitchen Timer
One you can carry around is great.

Your Imagination
Try a few different seasoning and cooking methods, until you find the ones you like. A little **seasoning** and **marinating** before cooking, just takes a little bit of **planning and time** and will add to your **enjoyment** and **satisfaction.**

Taste Tested Tips & Techniques

BEEF and VEAL: Cooking Suggestions

Shopping Tip:

Save some money by checking the meat department in your store for items **marked for quick sale.** These are meats that are near their 'sell by' dates. They are perfectly fine if you take them home and either **cook or freeze immediately.**

Best Preparation:

A good approach is to **do batches** of meat. I like to cut, trim and weigh them right after I bring them home. Then I **cook** a **batch** or **freeze** in marked bags. Once you get the habit you will **always have a supply** of meat ready.

If frozen, thaw. **Trim all visible fat** and if you haven't done this already, weigh RAW, cutting pieces to 3.75 oz.

Pre season and/or marinate 3-4 hours before cooking. Wash your hands and utensils carefully before and after. A great approach is to sprinkle on your beef seasoning and then **massage it** into the meat a little.

For a simple marinade that tastes great and is safe, use your **'Mom in a bottle' dressing.** The vinegar is a natural meat tenderizer so don't over marinate.

Best Cooking Methods.

Number One: Barbecue on the **gas grill** on medium **low heat** (250 degrees temperature on your BBQ) purchase a **cheap but loud** timer. Start out setting it for **5 minutes.** Warm the BBQ for 5 minutes. When the alarm goes off, **reset it** as you add your seasoned and marinated meat to the grill. **Turn every 5 minutes,** each time setting the timer before you turn the meat. Repeat until you get the desired doneness you like, trying not to over cook. **Be patient.**

Number Two: 'George Foreman Grill.' Most don't have a heat setting, just on or off. The **only control is time.** Use your timer and try different settings. Start with 2 minutes. Different cuts of meat are a little different, so once again **cook in batches and experiment** until you find the right setting for you. Write down the answer for next time. You will be able to easily **repeat the results.**

Appendix A   **REFERENCE: Helpful Recipes & Techniques**

Taste Tested Tips & Techniques

CHICKEN: Cooking Suggestions

Shopping Tip:

Buy frozen, skinless chicken breasts. You can find these in the 'all natural' and sometimes 'organic' variety. They are processed and dipped in water and **flash frozen**. So they are just as fresh, maybe fresher than the 'fresh' ones in the meat case. Price is reasonable as there is **very little waste**.

Best Preparation:

Once again, a good approach is to **do batches**. Start with **two chicken breasts**, which allowing for rotation, will give you enough (4 servings) for 2 days. I find that the frozen chicken breasts as they come in the package, are about the right weight when **cut in half** and trimmed.

Place a batch of **frozen chicken breasts** in a pan to thaw. I like to sprinkle them with a good 'poultry seasoning'.

Partially thaw.

Just thaw enough so that you can trim and cut them, but they are **still frozen enough** to **retain some moisture** from the freezing process. **Trim all visible fat** and weigh RAW cutting pieces to 3.75 oz. **Always wash your hands and utensils carefully.**

Best Cooking Methods.

Number One: You should start **barbecueing** on the **gas grill** on **medium low heat** (250 degrees) **before** completely thawed. This will result in **moister and more tender** chicken.

Use your cheap but loud timer. Start out setting it for 5 minutes. Warm the BBQ for 5 minutes. When the alarm goes off, **restart it as you add** your seasoned chicken breasts to the grill. Turn every 5 minutes, each time setting the timer **before you turn** the meat. (Less chance that you will forget and over-cook!) Repeat until you get the desired doneness you like, **trying not to over cook**. Be patient.

The best barbecuing secret? Go slow!

Number Two: Because of the slight tendency of the 'George Foreman Grill' to dry chicken out, **baking** is my next recommendation **for great chicken** results.

Best Preparation:

The same preparation as above **except** completely thaw the chicken pieces before baking. Once again, a good approach is to **do batches**. Baked chicken keeps well.

Use a **fresh baking dish** that is large enough to **avoid stacking** the chicken pieces. Line the bottom of the dish with fresh **baby spinach leaves**. A good heavy layer. Place seasoned chicken and top each piece with a thin slice of **fresh lemon**.

Cover with tin foil and bake at 375 for about 40 minutes. Ovens do vary, so **test** the chicken **the first time** to get the exact time, for the doneness you prefer. Write it down.

Number Three: Use the 'George Forman Grill,' much the same way that you did the beef grilling. With **a little practice** you will easily figure out the amount of time you need. Be careful to **avoid drying out** the chicken, by overcooking .

The great thing about this grill is, it removes excess fat. Not a lot of that in a properly trimmed chicken breast. Once you do figure out the correct time, it is **very repeatable** with George's 'lean mean grillin' machine. Write down your **cooking time**.

CHICKEN EGGS: Protein in a shell

Best Preparation.

Eggs are a source of **protein** you can utilize and said to be one of nature's most complete foods.

Studies have been done that would indicate that eggs as a source of **cholesterol** related problems is way **overblown**. If you are over concerned about cholesterol, a good optional approach is to use two egg whites for each egg yolk.

I think where eggs get a bad rap is from the most prevalent **method of preparation**... that would be 'fried'... don't!

Best Cooking Methods.

Cook your eggs by **boiling** or **poaching** and you are getting the beneficial inputs from eggs and minimizing the negative.

SEAFOOD: Low Fat Fish, Shellfish, Shrimp

Best Preparation.

Be careful to use very fresh or frozen varieties of the species listed in the HCG + 500 Seafood charts. Seafood is available in many fresh frozen varieties or you may have the opportunity to catch it your self.

Best Cooking Methods.

Seafood can be cooked the same as chicken, that would be **barbecue, bake** and **grill** and **in addition steamed**.

Seafood **cooks very quickly**, so once again some **testing** and experimenting when cooking it the first time, will serve you well.

Watch out for **sugar** in the seafood seasoning and sauces.

Seafood is a category of food that **can cause** your weight loss to **stall** or **diminish**. If you have that problem look at your menu records, if you suspect the seafood is the problem **cut back** or **eliminate** it for the **HCG + 500 Calorie** phase of treatment.

SUMMARY: Have Some Fun!

It helps to **keep your perspective**. You can do this! It is just a such **a short time** in your life and staying focused and giving it your best effort will really pay off with what can be **life changing** results and **very quickly** the pounds and inches will just melt away and it will all be worth it!

Just go for it!

Appendix A   **REFERENCE: Helpful Recipes & Techniques**

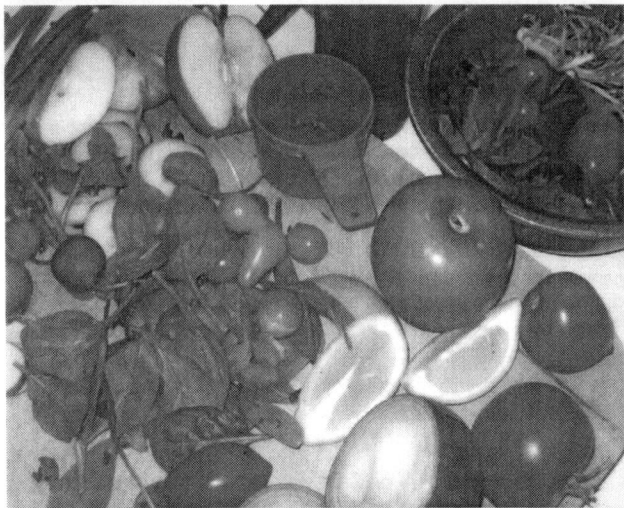

The Basic 'Go-To' Green Salad.

Summary of this Tested Recipe:

A basic green salad will normally be the foundation for a number of variations of basic salad recipes.

This recipe **covers the basics** and some additions to achieve the necessary variety and rotation needed for your **HCG + 500 Calorie** menu plan.

Making good **fresh and nutritious** salads with some **eye appeal** goes a long way toward keeping things **simple** and on **target**. Under 250 calories and filling.

You can use **any variety of apple** so experiment until you find a few favorites. Just changing from a sweet to a tart apple, not to mention **the color it adds**, can change the **flavor** and **taste** so you don't get bored.

Refrigerate apples as soon as you get them home. Store at 42-45 degrees for maximum crispy life.

The 'Apple ChickenSalad' shown here was created using the 'Go-To Green Salad' and adding crisp Gala Apples and skinless trimmed & grilled chicken breast and the 'Mom in a Bottle' Dressing recipe you just learned. Low Calories and very tasty.

What You Will Need:

Green Lettuce Mix
Organic & Fresh & Clean!
You can find a variety of these and they are normally reasonably priced and carefully washed and packaged

Baby Spinach Leaves
Rotation of your vegetables is a key. So you can easily substitute this vegetable choice for the lettuce.

Fresh & Crisp Apples
Any variety will work. Each one adds a variation of taste and eye appeal and even crispness. Have fun... experiment!

Fresh 'Organic' Lemon
You can eat a lemon everyday. I like to squeeze fresh lemon juice on my salads just before eating.

A bonus is the **lemon juice** keeps the apples from turning brown.

Your Choice of Protein
Use a variety, remembering to rotate the protein type, watch the Calories here!

Your 'Mom in a Bottle' Homemade Dressing
Experiment a little and customize this to your taste buds. Best to taste **test after applying** to your salad.

The Recipe:

2 Cups of Lettuce or Baby Spinach
Organic is best. Chop slightly just before preparing to help release the flavor.
(2 cups 42/22 Calories)

1 Medium Apple (Your Choice)
Organic is best. Core & Chop to bite sized. (70 Calories)

1/4 Cup 'Mom in a Bottle' Apple Cider Vinegar Dressing
Your custom Mix (2 oz. 10 Calories)

Optional Additions:
3.75 oz. Protein of Choice
Fat Free Chicken (85 Calories)
Low Fat Beef (185 Calories)
Low Fat Fish (80-110 Calories)

Juice 1/4 Fresh Lemon (optional)
0 Calories)

Taste Tested Tips & Techniques

Take a **handful of lettuce** or **baby leaf spinach** and roll it up and cut just before you are ready to eat your salad. This **releases the flavor** of the greenery. Can you smell it?

It is best to mix just the amount of salad **you are going to eat** and make it up fresh each time. Just takes a few minutes and it will taste **fresher, crispier and more flavorful**.

Here's What You Do:

Lightly chop **lettuce** or **baby spinach**. Place in a shallow bowl or dish. Add your choice of **cut up apples** and your choice of **meat** with all visible fat removed.

Shake up your **'Mom in a Bottle'** homemade dressing and **add to salad**. Toss well and enjoy.

(165-240 Calories Depending on protein choice)

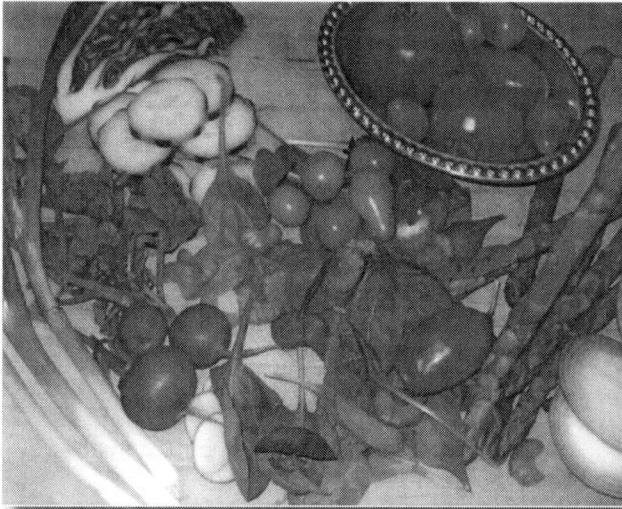

The 'Veggie Team'

Your 'Veggie Team' Substitutes

Summary: How to use your 'bench.'

You have your meat cooked.
You have your 'Mom in a Bottle' dressing
You have fixed a 'go to' green salad.

Now what?

Let's review. Making good **fresh and nutritious** salads with some **eye appeal** goes a long way toward keeping things simple and on target and **under 250 calories**.

You can use **any variety of apple**. Want to know how to get the rest of the **veggie team** involved, to change the flavor and taste, so you don't get bored?

Check out the ideas below.

Taste Tested Tips & Techniques

ASPARAGUS (4 oz. = 25 Calories)

Cooked: Steam or boil.
Use as a main vegetable instead of salad.
'Mom in a Bottle' Dressing is great with this.

CABBAGE (1 cup = 27 Calories)

Raw: cut like 'cole slaw' add chopped apple and 'Mom in a Bottle' Dressing
Cooked: Bake with chicken or veal

CELERY (1 cup = 17 Calories)

Salad: Chop and mix with chopped apple for a fresh crunchy, crunchy salad. Make dressing add 1/4 cup pureed cottage cheese (58 Calories) and 'Mom in a Bottle.'
By the stalk: Stuff with cotttage cheese and a dash of dill weed. Great for a snack.

CUCUMBERS (1 cup = 16 Calories)

Raw: Slice and put in a bowl of Mom in a Bottle dressing. Chill well. You can also make a cucumber and apple salad.

ONIONS (1 small = 29 Calories)

Grilled: The 'George Foreman Grill' works great.
You can add these to the grill at the same time as your steak and grill together. Adds a nice flavor. Changes the cooking.
Baked: Bake in the oven (350 for 75 minutes) and eat with seasoning, salt and pepper or dressing.

RED RADISHES (1 cup = 30 Calories)

Raw: I like to slice these very thin and salt and eat like potato chips. Filling and very low Calorie.

SPINACH, RAW/COOKED (1 cup = 11/41 Calories)

Raw: Use as a salad substitute.
Cooked: Bake with your chicken.
Steamed: Use as your main vegetable

TOMATOES, Cherry (1 cup = 27 Calories)

Raw: A great low Calorie snack, that is oozing with nutrients.
Cooked: Puree and add to organic beef or chicken broth. Makes a nice soup. Great on a cold day.

TOMATOES, Mediium (1 medium = 35 Calories)

Raw: A great low Calorie snack, that is oozing with nutrients.
Cooked: Puree and add to organic beef or chicken broth. Makes a nice soup. Great on a cold day.

NOTE: Tomatoes are a potential weight loss staller!

Where's the LETTUCE?

The Lettuce is a star!

See the 'Go to Green Salad'

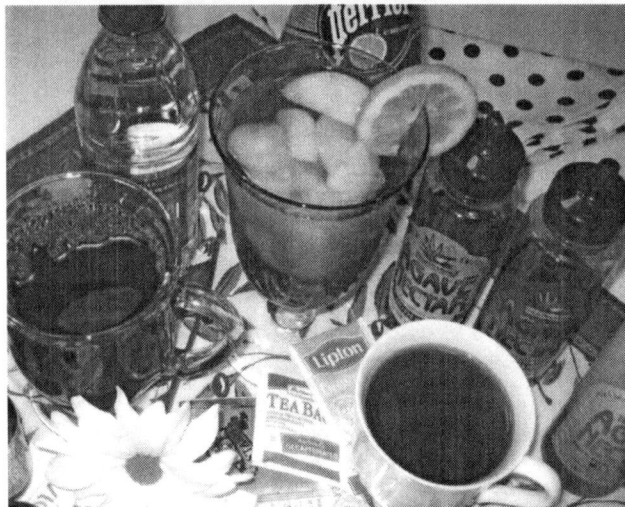

Water... Water... Everywhere? What else to drink?

Water, Water...Not Everywhere?

Summary: 'Variations on a Theme'

No Limit on Approved Drinks.

Let's review what is **approved** by the good doctor **without restrictions:**

- All types of Coffees & Teas
- Pure Mineral Water
- Pure Fresh Water
- Daily Fresh Squeezed Lemon Juice

Your fluid intake should be **at least 68 oz.** a day.

Drinking hot or cold liquids does help **curb** and **control** your **appetite.**

Check out the ideas below.

Taste Tested Tips & Techniques

HOT DRINKS:

HOT COFFEE:
Organic whenever possible, decaf or the regular kind.

Additives:
Natural sweeteners, Stevia is actually available in lots of flavors. They have a four flavor small portable assortment you can carry around. Sorry, only 1 tablespoon of milk a day.

Coffee is a **'diuretic.'** Doctor talk for frequent bladder emptying. So be sure to drink plenty of other liquids.

HOT TEAS:
Organic whenever possible, decaf or the regular kind. Teas also claim to have other desirable benefits. Check the labels.

Additives:
Natural sweeteners, Stevia is actually available in lots of Flavors. They have a four flavor small portable assortment you can carry around. Sorry, only 1 tablespoon of milk a day.

Tea is an **'acid.'** Tannic acid to be precise. Some find it upsetting on an empty stomach. Also a **'diuretic.'** So be sure to drink plenty of other liquids.

HOT CHOCOLATE:
Actually made with hot water and 'chocolate' flavored Stevia.

Additives:
Sorry, only 1 tablespoon of milk a day.

Some find this good and add some other flavored Stevia to customize it. Helps if you are a chocolate craver. I am not a Stevia lover, but start with about five drops and experiment a little.

COLD DRINKS:

ICED COFFEE:
Organic whenever possible, decaf or the regular kind. A nice refreshing drink on a hot summer day!

Additives:
Natural sweeteners, Stevia is actually available in lots of flavors. They have a four flavor small portable assortment you can carry around. Sorry, only 1 tablespoon of milk a day.

Coffee is a **'diuretic.'** Doctor talk for frequent bladder emptying. So be sure to drink plenty of other liquids.

ICED TEA:
Organic whenever possible, decaf or the regular kind. 'Sun tea' is my favorite way of brewing. Refrigerate until nice and frosty.

Additives:
Natural sweeteners, Stevia is actually is available in lots of flavors. They have a four flavor small portable assortment you can carry around. Sorry, only 1 tablespoon of milk a day.

Tea is an **'acid.'** Tannic acid to be precise. Some find it upsetting on an empty stomach. Also a **'diuretic.'** So be sure to drink plenty of other liquids.

ICED COLD LEMONADE:
Fresh squeezed Organic Lemon juice added to water or mineral water. Refrigerate until nice and frosty.

Additives:
Natural sweeteners, Stevia is available in fruit flavors. Agave Nectar, is now flavored, as well. You can make a fake strawberry lemonade. Later you add real strawberries as you finish your **HCG + 500 Calorie** phase.

Appendix B:
'Charting & Navigating'

"How many promising careers have been ruined by excessive fat; how many lives have been shortened?"

Dr. A.T.W. Simeons

Defeat OBESITY...Forever!

The HCG Assisted 500 Calorie Weight Loss Cure

Appendix B   'Charting & Navigating'

Going, Going... Gone!

Now we are going to **track your progress** and record and graph your weight loss.

You will find **copies** of all of the **forms** shown in the pages that follow. You will be using them to transfer your results from your daily menu planners and daily keep track of your **vanishing 'pounds and inches.'**

"Now we are going to track your progress and record and graph your weight loss."

Vanishing Pounds & Inches

	Date: 12/31	Date: 1/1	Date: 1/2	Date: 1/3	Date: 1/4	Date: 1/5	Date: 1/6	Date: 1/7	Date: 1/8	Date: 1/9	Date: 1/10	Date: 1/11	Date: 1/12
Weight Forward	247	247	238	235.5	230.5	230.0	228.5	228.0	225.5	223.5	223.5	223.5	222.0
A.M. Weight	247	238	235.5	230.5	230.0	228.5	228.0	225.5	223.5	223.5	223.5	222.0	222.0
POUNDS LOST	0	9	2.5	5.0	.5	1.5	.5	4.5	2.0	0	0	1.5	0
TOTAL LOST	0	9	11.5	16.5	17.0	18.5	19.0	23.5	25.5	25.5	25.5	27.0	27.0
Notes:	1st day				5 days					10 days	Apple Day "stall"		

Health Measurements

	Date: 12/31	Date: 1/1	Date: 1/2	Date: 1/3	Date: 1/4	Date: 1/5	Date: 1/6	Date: 1/7	Date: 1/8	Date: 1/9	Date: 1/10	Date: 1/11	Date: 1/12	
Blood Sugar	300	219	259	228	214	203	225	196	184	182	184	191	164	18

"...transfer your results from your daily menu planners and daily keep track of your vanishing 'pounds and inches.'"

Keeping it Simple.

You will note that the **form above** covers 20 days, or as the doctor would put it, one 'course' of HCG treatment.

Don't be intimidated by this form, it is really **simple** and takes but a few **minutes** to complete. Just start at the upper left corner. Fill in the date. Under **'Weight Forward'** write today's weight. Moving straight down fill in **'A.M. Weight.'** Note: On your **first** day, those first two **weight numbers** will be **the same**.

Okay, move straight down to **'Pounds Lost'** and then **'Total Lost,'** once again on the first day, both of these will be the same... that would be zero. Keep going down and make any **'Notes'** and add any personal **'Health Measurements'** or **'RX Records'** (you know... prescriptions) that **you and your doctor** have determined are needed on a **daily basis**. That's all there is to it.

"...it is really simple and takes but a few minutes to complete."

On the **second day** the previous days **'A.M. Weight'** moves **over and up** to the **'Weight Forward'** box. Then write in **today's weight** and **subtract** to get the **'Pounds Lost.'** To arrive at the **'Total Lost'** you simply **add** todays **'Pounds Lost'** to yesterdays **'Total Lost'** which will give you the **'fun number'**...your pounds lost. Also don't forget to record the other **measurements** you are tracking.

CHARTS

&

RECORD KEEPING

CHARTS & RECORD KEEPING

Vanishing Pounds & Inches

Date:	Date:	Date:	Date:	Date:	Date:	Date:	Date:	Date:	Date:	Date:	Date:	Date:	Date:	Date:	Date:
Weight Forward	Weight Forward	Weight Forward	Weight Forward	Weight Forward	Weight Forward	Weight Forward	Weight Forward	Weight Forward	Weight Forward	Weight Forward	Weight Forward	Weight Forward	Weight Forward	Weight Forward	Weight Forward
A.M. Weight	A.M. Weight	A.M. Weight	A.M. Weight	A.M. Weight	A.M. Weight	A.M. Weight	A.M. Weight	A.M. Weight	A.M. Weight	A.M. Weight	A.M. Weight	A.M. Weight	A.M. Weight	A.M. Weight	A.M. Weight
POUNDS LOST	POUNDS LOST	POUNDS LOST	POUNDS LOST	POUNDS LOST	POUNDS LOST	POUNDS LOST	POUNDS LOST	POUNDS LOST	POUNDS LOST	POUNDS LOST	POUNDS LOST	POUNDS LOST	POUNDS LOST	POUNDS LOST	POUNDS LOST
TOTAL LOST	TOTAL LOST	TOTAL LOST	TOTAL LOST	TOTAL LOST	TOTAL LOST	TOTAL LOST	TOTAL LOST	TOTAL LOST	TOTAL LOST	TOTAL LOST	TOTAL LOST	TOTAL LOST	TOTAL LOST	TOTAL LOST	TOTAL LOST
Notes:	Notes:	Notes:	Notes:	Notes:	Notes:	Notes:	Notes:	Notes:	Notes:	Notes:	Notes:	Notes:	Notes:	Notes:	Notes:

Optional Health Measurements

Date:	Date:	Date:	Date:	Date:	Date:	Date:	Date:	Date:	Date:	Date:	Date:	Date:	Date:
Blood SUGAR	Blood SUGAR	Blood SUGAR	Blood SUGAR	Blood SUGAR	Blood SUGAR	Blood SUGAR	Blood SUGAR	Blood SUGAR	Blood SUGAR	Blood SUGAR	Blood SUGAR	Blood SUGAR	Blood SUGAR
Blood PRESSURE	Blood PRESSURE	Blood PRESSURE	Blood PRESSURE	Blood PRESSURE	Blood PRESSURE	Blood PRESSURE	Blood PRESSURE	Blood PRESSURE	Blood PRESSURE	Blood PRESSURE	Blood PRESSURE	Blood PRESSURE	Blood PRESSURE

RX Records	RX Records	RX Records	RX Records	RX Records	RX Records	RX Records	RX Records	RX Records

ISBN 978-0-9800641-8-6

Vanishing Pounds & Inches

Date: | Date: | Date: | Date: | Date: | Date: | Date: | Date: | Date: | Date: | Date: | Date: | Date: | Date: | Date:

- Weight Forward
- A.M. Weight
- POUNDS LOST
- TOTAL LOST
- Notes:

Optional Health Measurements

Date: | Date: | Date: | Date: | Date: | Date: | Date: | Date: | Date: | Date: | Date: | Date: | Date: | Date: | Date:

- Blood SUGAR
- Blood PRESSURE
- RX Records

Vanishing Pounds & Inches

Date: | Date: | Date: | Date: | Date: | Date: | Date: | Date: | Date: | Date: | Date: | Date: | Date: | Date: | Date: | Date: | Date: | Date:

Weight Forward (blank cells across)

A.M. Weight (blank cells across)

POUNDS LOST (blank cells across)

TOTAL LOST (blank cells across)

Notes: (blank cells across)

Optional Health Measurements

Date: | Date: | Date: | Date: | Date: | Date: | Date: | Date: | Date:

Blood SUGAR (blank cells across)

Blood PRESSURE (blank cells across)

RX Records (blank cells across)

Section Four: **'Charting & Navigating'**

Your 'Poof it's Gone' Chart.

One of the funest and most **exciting things** you can do to keep **motivated** and **on course** is to transfer your pounds & inches **numbers,** to the chart **shown below.**

If you are doing it right you will most likely experience what all of the HCG Alums experience. That would be **dramatic** and rapid **weight loss,** followed by, of course, disappearing **inches.** A slight lag between the two is perfectly normal.

As I have shared before, **I lost 22 pounds** in the first **7 days**, so brace yourself.

"One of the funnest and most exciting things you can do to keep motivated..."

"...dramatic and rapid weight loss, followed by, of course, disappearing inches..."

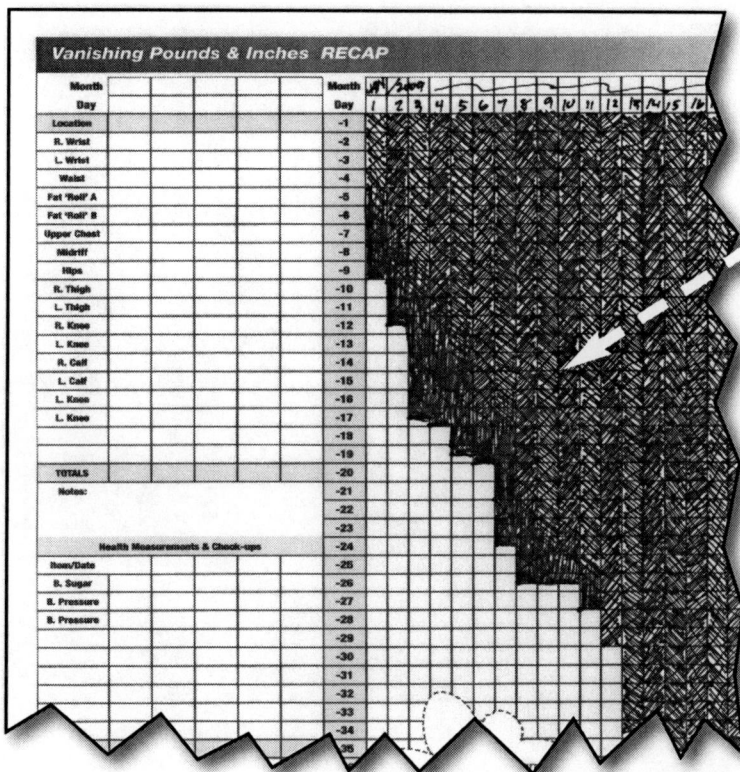

Color in the POUNDS as You Lose Them!

These are the Actual Pounds I lost on the HCG + 500 Calorie Diet Phase

The Proof is in the 'Poofing.'

Here is **how to use** this 'Poof' recap chart.

"...each box represents one pound lost..."

Look in the center and you will see a series of **numbers** from **'-1'** to **'-47'** that is the number of accumulative **pounds** you have **lost.** That figure comes from the **'Total Lost'** box on your **'Vanishing Pounds & Inches'** form that we just covered.

On this form, you just **color** in the number of vertical boxes, **each box** represents **one pound lost**, to graphically show your pounds lost. It's that fun and simple.

Be sure to **record the dates** carefully, of course, and utilize the other optional parts of the form to track your **measurements**, **medical conditions** or **medications**.

RECAP Pounds & Inches

Month						Month	Day																										
Day						Day																												
Location						-1																												
R. Wrist						-2																												
L. Wrist						-3																												
Waist						-4																												
Fat 'Roll' A						-5																												
Fat 'Roll' B						-6																												
Upper Chest						-7																												
Midriff						-8																												
Hips						-9																												
R. Thigh						-10																												
L. Thigh						-11																												
R. Knee						-12																												
L. Knee						-13																												
R. Calf						-14																												
L. Calf						-15																												
L. Knee						-16																												
L. Knee						-17																												
						-18																												
						-19																												
TOTALS						-20																												
Notes:						-21																												
						-22																												
						-23																												
Health Measurements & Check-ups						-24																												
Item/Date						-25																												
B. Sugar						-26																												
B. Pressure						-27																												
B. Pressure						-28																												
						-29																												
						-30																												
						-31																												
						-32																												
						-33																												
						-34																												
RX/Quit Date						-35																												
						-36																												
						-37																												
						-38																												
						-39																												
						-40																												
						-41																												
						-42																												
						-43																												
						-44																												
						-45																												
						-46																												
						-47																												

Your Very Own
"Poof it's gone!"
CHART

RECAP Pounds & Inches

Month						Month	Day
Day						Day	
Location						-1	
R. Wrist						-2	
L. Wrist						-3	
Waist						-4	
Fat 'Roll' A						-5	
Fat 'Roll' B						-6	
Upper Chest						-7	
Midriff						-8	
Hips						-9	
R. Thigh						-10	
L. Thigh						-11	
R. Knee						-12	
L. Knee						-13	
R. Calf						-14	
L. Calf						-15	
L. Knee						-16	
L. Knee						-17	
						-18	
						-19	
TOTALS						-20	
Notes:						-21	
						-22	
						-23	
Health Measurements & Check-ups						-24	
Item/Date						-25	
B. Sugar						-26	
B. Pressure						-27	
B. Pressure						-28	
						-29	
						-30	
						-31	
						-32	
						-33	
						-34	
RX/Quit Date						-35	
						-36	
						-37	
						-38	
						-39	
						-40	
						-41	
						-42	
						-43	
						-44	
						-45	
						-46	
						-47	

Your Very Own "Poof it's gone!" CHART

Section One: Write Your VICTORY Story Here!

Case History:

HCG Alumni

Paste
YOUR

BEFORE

Photo
HERE

BEFORE HCG:

Weight:
Waist:

Medical Concerns:

Number of RX:
RX Cost:

AFTER HCG:

Weight:
Waist:

Medical Concerns:

Number of RX:
RX Cost:

Paste
YOUR

AFTER

Photo
HERE

Your Story:

Case History:

HCG Alumni

Paste
YOUR

BEFORE

Photo
HERE

BEFORE HCG:

Weight:
Waist:

Medical Concerns:

Number of RX:
RX Cost:

AFTER HCG:

Weight:
Waist:

Medical Concerns:

Number of RX:
RX Cost:

Paste
YOUR

AFTER

Photo
HERE

Your Story:

Appendix C:
'Trouble Shooting'

"Failure is simply the opportunity to begin again... more intelligently."

Henry Ford

Defeat OBESITY...Forever!

The HCG Assisted 500 Calorie Weight Loss Cure

Appendix C: **Troubleshooting: INTRODUCTION**

"The purpose... ... is to help you solve any problems..."

Troubleshooting Tips & Techniques Summary.

The purpose of this section is to help you solve any problems you may encounter. Dr. Simeons plan **works** as advertised, but it is precise and needs to be followed carefully and exactly. Below is a short **summary** of the contents of this section.

Food for Thought.

Understanding why we can, and do have a difficult time, struggling with obesity.

5 Things That Can Sidetrack Your Efforts.

A short list of common **pitfalls** to avoid. They are listed in no particular order since each of us has our own number one issue. Sometime it helps to see them in print.

"Sometimes it helps to see them in print."

Forget the 'Guilt Trip.' Shop Smart.

How to be a smart grocery shopper and avoid those shopping issues. Ever wonder how you end up with a bunch of high priced **'junk food'** in your cupboard? In the grocery business they call that 'merchandising.' I spent years in that business and I have laid out the antidote for you. I think a key ingredient in weight control is your shopping **strategy**. Here's how to gain the upperhand over grocery guilt trips.

Understanding Weight Plateaus.

This is **natural** and likely to happen. No need to panic, Dr. Simeons to the rescue. A short check list for you and a description of what this is all about.

"The antidote for plateau panic."

Dr. Simeons Pacifier the 'Apple Day'

The antidote for 'plateau panic.'

Check Your Exercise & Rest Cycles.

Very important to get proper rest and moderate exercise, avoid stressful workouts. Rember your 'fat facts (see page 25) extreme excercising does **not** increase your loss of 'warehouse fat' since it burns your 'dynamic' fat, which is promptly regained.

No Sugar or Starch: The 2 Pound Limit.

The Answer: **'Steak Day'** & Understanding **'Protein Deficiency.'**
Bonus: Another Steak Day Variation

"These can trip you up, ladies."

Caution: Bathing & Grooming Products

These these can trip you up, ladies: Cosmetics, Massages & Manicures.

Some Approved Products:

Table C-1: Alternative and approved products.
Don't panic, you can do this.

Back of the Book.

The Victory Collection of HCG Diet books & other **GreatNewsPress.com** books.

TROUBLE SHOOTING:

TIPS & TECHNIQUES

TROUBLE SHOOTING:

Appendix C: **Trouble Shooting: TIPS & TECHNIQUES**

"... the avearge american eats 3000 Calories daily!"

Food... for Thought?

According to recent published estimates, the **average american** eats **3000 Calories** daily! Recall the little **'Nutrition Labels'** on food products? They normally use **2000 Calories as an average reference.** Apparently **'too much'** is average.

That's **how we got into trouble,** packing away all of that **fat in our warehouse.** An **extra 1500 Calories per day** will add about **12 lbs a year** to our 'storage facility.'

Spoiled by 'Success'

"Apparently too much ... is average!"

Remember old Albert, who said, "...insanity is **repeating** the **same thing** over and over and **expecting different results...**" Our health and obesity problems grew out of our 'success' in finding and consuming **too many Calories**... which adds to our girth and **requires more**... you guessed it... CALORIES.

5 Things That Can Sidetrack Your Efforts.

You will find more about these pitfalls in **this section,** but it won't hurt to take a quick look at the more **common ways,** that your carefully laid **plans can go astray.**

These are in no particular order, but are especiallly **important** throughout the diet.

"Not all Calories are out in the open..."

- **Poor Discipline**
- **Losing Track of Daily Calories**
- **Portion Control**
- **Food Choices**
- **Hidden 'Sugars & Starches'**

Forget the 'Guilt Trip!' Shop Smart.

I am **not** trying to send you on a guilt trip. But I am **sending you on a 'smart' grocery shopping trip.** So awareness of the 'enemy' lurking in those food aisles is a very prudent consideration.

Here are a few **words of wisdom,** learned when I worked in the **grocery business.** Grocers know that **shopper studies show** ways to increase profit and volume.

"...insanity is repeating the same thing over and over and expecting different results..."

- **Slower Shoppers Spend More**
- **Hungry Shoppers Spend More**
- **Highest Priced Items Sell Best at 'Eye level'**
- **Feature 'Convenience' & 'Comfort Foods' Prominently**

Why are these things important? Simply put, the **quicker** you shop and the more **disciplined** and **organized** you are, the **more efficiently you will shop,** and I believe, you will also be a **healthier** shopper.

Eat first then shop, use a **shopping list,** shop the **outside aisles** for **perishables first** (Fruits, vegetables and meats) **avoid convenience foods** (think highly processed & expensive) Watch out for **'comfort' foods** (think sugar and starch) **Read the labels** and if it has any **sugar or starch in the ingredients**... don't buy it. **These things are critical** for victory and overall, in my opinion, a good lifestyle.

A final thought on this topic... be extra careful in those big 'food warehouses.'

| Appendix C: | Trouble Shooting: TIPS & TECHNIQUES |

Problem:

" I seem to be 'stuck'... not gaining or losing...

What do I do?

Understanding 'Weight Plateaus.'

If you have **followed the plan carefully**, hitting little pauses in your weight loss is **nothing** to be concerned about, There are **several possible causes**.

This is where your careful **record keeping**, yes, the ones I have been harping about, become an invaluable tool. Also a plateau is more likely during the **HCG + 500 Calorie** phase. Dr. Simeons reassures us, that it is simply a normal sequence of events. He also indicates that if you **stay the course** eventually you will break the plateau and continue to lose weight normally.

A plateau seems to be inevitable if you start out losing weight very quickly... and most of us do. Assuming you have not committed any dietary errors, if you are **stalled for 4-6 days**, here is what you should do;

Solutions:

"An 'apple-day' begins at lunch and continues until just before lunch of the following day..."

　　1) Check your menu plan for any errors.
　　2) Check your seasoning, etc. for any hidden sugars or starches.
　　3) Have you eaten any tomatoes, oranges or seafood?

You can consult with your doctor, but if **everything checks out** okay, you are probably having, what I like to call, a **'normal adjustment plateau.'** Here's why.

As you burn Calories from your stored fat, the **supporting tissues**, blood vessels, etc., that exist solely to service, that warehouse fat, remain. In a few days they will **be fully absorbed** into your body and your downward weight march will resume.

The **bonus** here, is that all of the vitamins and minerals, etc. in those tissues, is absorbed into **back into your system**, along with the **fat** and the **nutrients** in it.

"...The 'apple-day' produces a gratifying loss of weight on the following day, chiefly due to the elimination of water..."

The **exception** of course, is if you are about at the end of your HCG plan, and your supply of **warehouse fat** is **exhausted**. Consult with **your doctor**, to see for sure.

Dr. Simeons Pacifier... the 'Apple Day'

"An 'apple-day' begins at lunch and continues until just before lunch of the following day. The patients are given **six large apples** and are told to eat one whenever they feel the desire though six apples is the **maximum** allowed.

During an apple-day **no** other **food** or **liquids except plain water** are allowed and of water, they may only drink, if eating an apple still leaves them thirsty. Just enough to quench an uncomfortable thirst,

Most patients feel no need for water and are **quite happy** with their six apples.

"Be sure to get adequete rest and enough sleep to avoid affecting your weigh loss..."

The **apple-day** produces a gratifying loss of weight on the following day, chiefly due to the **elimination of water.** This water is not regained when the patients resume their normal 500-Calorie diet at lunch, and on the following days they continue to **lose weight** satisfactorily."

Check Your Exercise & Rest Cycles.

The good doctor does not see a huge benefit in rigorous exercise and recommends that **moderate** exercise is fine. Remember, you are targeting your 'stored fat.' Not the 'dynamic fat,' that your body taps into when stressed, and then replaces.

Not getting **adequate rest** and enough sleep will negatively affect your weight loss.

Appendix C: **Trouble Shooting TIPS & TECHNIQUES**

Problem:

"I am over the 2 pound limit on my weight setting phase...

...How Can I Fix That?"

Solutions:

"A 'steak day..."

"... fast all day. No breakfast, no lunch, then for dinner eat a huge lean beef steak..."

No Sugar No Starch & The 2 pound Limit.

A critical part of your success in resetting your body's s weight management system to your new and improved weight is the infamous '2 pound limit.'

If you exceed the 2 pound **gain limit**, you must immediately take corrective action.

The 'Steak Day' is the Answer.

Here's the **answer**. You fast all day. No breakfast, no lunch, then for dinner eat a huge lean beef steak. What do I mean by huge? 12 to 16 ounces.

With your steak, you may have an apple and some tomatoes (or organic, no sugar ketchup) Remember to drink your liquids without limit. Cold or hot drinks curb hunger.

You will probably find yourself, up emptying your bladder more than usual that night. You will be rewarded in the morning. 'Poof' **the extra pounds** will be gone.

I found that I needed **one** steak day a week to keep within the 2 lb. limit, during the 21 day stretch. So don't panic if you need a 'steak day' to get back on track. It's normal.

You are now in charge of your body's weight management system, and you never have to go back to the obesity lifestyle' again. You are probably healthier as a result.

Protein Deficiency 'hunger - edema' Explained.

Once again, read what the good doctor has to say, about a common misconception.

"During treatment the patient has been only just above the verge of protein deficiency and has had the advantage of protein being fed back into his system from the break-down of fatty tissue. Once the treatment is over there is no more HCG in the body and this process no longer takes place. Unless an **adequate** amount of **protein** is eaten as soon as the treatment is over, **protein deficiency** is bound to develop, and this inevitably causes the marked retention of water known as **hunger - edema**.

"Unless an adequate amount of protein is eaten as soon as the treatment is over, protein deficiency is bound to develop..."

The Treatment is Very Simple. Steak Day Variation.

The patient is told to eat **two eggs** for **breakfast** and a **huge steak** for **lunch** and **dinner** followed by a large helping of **cheese** and to phone through the weight the next morning. When these instructions are followed a stunned voice is heard to report that **two lbs.** have **vanished overnight**, that the ankles are normal but that sleep was disturbed, owing to an extraordinary need **to pass large quantities of water**.

The patient having learned this lesson usually has no further trouble."

(Note: This is just another version of the infamous 'steak day.')

www.HCGVictoryToolKit.com & www.HCGDietVictoryPlanner.com

Check our websites for updates, information and additional resources.

CAUTION: Bathing & Grooming Products

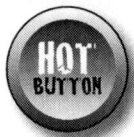

"Most women find it hard to believe that fats, oils, creams and ointments applied to the skin are absorbed and interfere..."

The 'Midas Touch'... Not Exactly!

One of the effects of **HCG** in your system is a **hypersensitivity** to sugars, starches, oils and fats. As surprising as it sounds, when it comes to oils & fats, this extends to **even touching** or rubbing them into your skin!

Here's an excerpt from Doctor Simeons on the subject.

> "When no dietary error is elicited we turn to cosmetics. Most women find it hard to believe that fats, oils, creams and ointments applied to the skin are absorbed and interfere with weight reduction by HCG just as if they had been eaten.
>
> This almost **incredible sensitivity** to even such very minor increases in nutritional intake is **a peculiar feature** of the HCG method.
>
> For instance, we find that persons who habitually handle organic fats, such as workers in beauty parlors, masseurs, butchers, etc. never show what we consider a satisfactory loss of weight unless they can avoid fat coming into contact with their skin."

Wow!

So that means, during the **relatively short time** that you are ingesting the HCG hormone, you need to studiously **avoid any oils or fats either eaten or applied** to **your body**... and yes... the same rules apply to **men** or **anyone on HCG**.

Here's a little more **specific advice** on the 'cosmetics' question from the doctor.

"We are particularly averse to those modern cosmetics which contain hormones..."

> "We are particularly averse to those modern cosmetics which contain hormones, as any interference with endocrine regulations during treatment must be absolutely avoided. Many women whose skin has in the course of years become adjusted to the use of fat containing cosmetics find that their skin gets dry as soon as they stop using them. In such cases we permit the use of **plain mineral oil**, which has no nutritional value."

> "We do permit the use of **lipstick, powder** and such lotions as are entirely **free of fatty substances**. We also allow brilliantine to be used on the hair but it must not be rubbed into the scalp. Obviously sun-tan oil is prohibited."

Times Have Changed... Products Also.

Since Dr. Simeons era there exists an increased awareness of the residual effects of products that come in contact with our skin. In fact some entire 'cosmetic' product lines exist primarily due to the sensitivity of their clients to various ingredients.

"...you should find it easier to obtain products that are 'HCG friendly' and contain no fats or oils."

The bottom line of all of this is **you should find it easier** to obtain products that are 'HCG friendly' and contain no fats or oils. So just like you should do when you look for spices and condiments... **read the ingredients** for the real story.

You may want to do **some special shopping** to get you by. See the short list on the next page for some general ideas and some **brand names** that are **safe.**

Appendix C: **CAUTION: Bathing & Grooming Products**

Massages.

This is another area of **potential problems** that is often not considered. Most massages use oils and lotions which **can stall your weight loss** and even result in weight gain. Doctor Simeons has some sage advice in that area.

"I never allow any kind of massage during treatment. It is entirely unnecessary and merely disturbs a very delicate process which is going on in the tissues.

"I never allow any kind of massage during treatment. It is entirely unnecessary and merely disturbs a very delicate process which is going on in the tissues."

Few indeed are the masseurs and masseuses who can resist the temptation to knead and hammer abnormal fat deposits. In the course of rapid reduction it is sometimes possible to pick up a fold of skin which has not yet had time to adjust itself, as it always does under HCG, to the changed figure.

This fold contains its normal subcutaneous fat and may be almost an inch thick. It is one of the main objects of the HCG treatment to keep that fat there. Patients and their masseurs do not always understand this and give this fat a working-over. I have seen such patients who were as black and blue as if they had received a sound thrashing."

Want to know how he really feels? Read this.

"How **anyone in his right mind** is able to believe that fatty tissue can be shifted mechanically or be made to vanish by squeezing is beyond my comprehension. The only effect obtained is severe bruising. The torn tissue then forms scars, and these slowly contract making the fatty tissue even harder and more unyielding."

Okay doctor, we get the picture. Time to **cancel or postpone** that massage.

Table C-1 Bathing & Beauty Products	
Product	**Safe Brands & Suggestions**
Bathing Soaps	Dial, Ivory, Zest or Other 'Oil Free' Soaps
Cosmetics	Any 'Oil Free' Product. Use the Minimum.
Cosmetic Removers	'Oil Free' brands or 'Witch Hazel'
Deodorants	Use natural or organic chemical free products
Hair Products	Check ingredients. Excercise caution on scalp.
Lipsticks & Balms	Minimize use during HCG + 500 Calorie Phase
Lotions & Potions	For dry skin Mineral Oil used very sparingly.
Sun Tan/Sun Screen	'Oil Free' products. Mineral Oil. Minimize or eliminate.
Toothpaste	Any 'Sugar Free' brand or Baking Soda

"...exercise caution, minimize their use when on HCG, read the labels and use good old 'common sense."

One Final Thought.

Ladies and gentlemen, you can usually use your regular products, without a problem, as long as you exercise caution, minimize their use when on HCG, read the labels and use good old **'common sense.'** Just keep the good doctor's warnings in mind!

Appendix C: **HCG Victory Collection BOOKS**

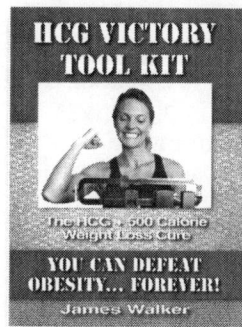

'HCG Victory Tool Kit'
©2009

'HCG Victory TOOL KIT'

A **comprehensive** and **easy to understand** guide for successfully winning your war with obesity. Clearly and carefully constructed to provide **maximum** help with a **minimum** of frustration. The book is really **four books in one** and indispensable.

It contains a complete road map and all of the food tables and recipes you need to succeed. Includes a generous supply of forms to plan, record and track your weight loss for the critical, **'HCG + 500 Calorie'** and **'No Sugar No Starch'** phases. A **bonus** is a completely new presentation of Doctor Simeons manuscript in an easier to read and understand **format**, with added table of contents and diagrams.

If you are serious about the HCG weight loss plan this is absolutely **the best book**.

204 pages (8.25 x 11.0 inches) **ISBN 978-0-9800641-7-9**

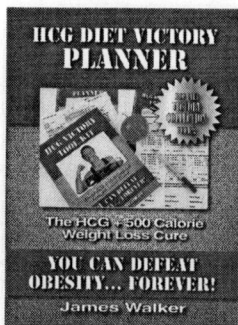

HCG Diet
Victory Planner
©2010

'HCG DIET Victory PLANNER'

By popular demand, book 2 in the Victory Collection a **companion volume** for use with the **'HCG Victory Tool Kit'** Emphasis is on weight setting & time saving.

All of the suggested menus and instructions for the **'No Sugar or Starch'** weight setting step are supplied. You will find **already filled out EZPLan™ menu plans** in 6 day sets. Use the plans as is or customize them. Bonus review of HCG + 500 Calorie step **plus** an important new report on the science of 'metabolic profiling.'

The sets of 6 day plans come in 1200 to 2600 Calories in 100 Calorie increments! **Just pick a menu and go.** In additon a generous supply of all of the blank menu plans, charts and forms, are also included! Bonus section on 'metabolic blueprints.'

If you want a **'turn-key' solution** for your HCG weight loss plan and a proven track to run on, then this book is the addition you need to your **'Victory Collection.'**

202 pages (8.25 x 11.0 inches) **ISBN 978-0-9800641-8-6**

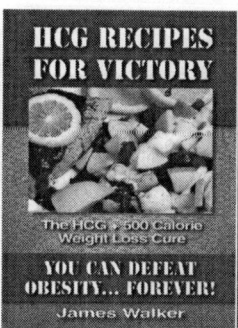

Super Simeons
'Recipes for
Victory'
©2010

'Super Simeons™ HCG DIET Victory RECIPES'

A **full color companion volume** for use with the **'HCG Victory Collection'**

A special collection of recipes for use with both the **'HCG + 500 Calorie'** and the **'No Sugar or Starch'** steps, as well as plenty of **'Return to Earth'** recipes for that trip back to **your new normal**. Full of mouth-watering **delicious** and **nutritious** recipes presented in eye appealing **full color!** Features the modular 'food element' concept introduced in the HCG Diet Victory Planner, EZPlans™ This facilitates expanding and including the whole family in your meal planning and preparation.

Allowances for all **metabolic** & nutritional profile types for you 'metabolic typers.'

If you want **a library of recipes** for your HCG weight loss plan and your **new body** and **lifestyle**, then add this **super recipe book** to your **'Victory Collection.'**

100 pages (8.5 x 11.0 inches) **ISBN 978-0-9800641-9-3**

Appendix C: INSPIRATIONAL BOOKS by GreatNewsPress.Com

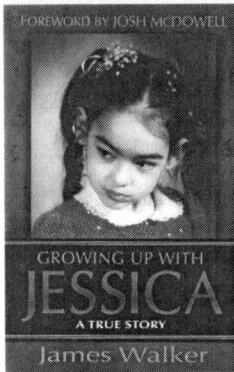

The 'Growing Up with JESSICA, Second Edition'

A **moving and inspirational true story**, told clearly and passionately by Jessica's father. Part mystery, part tragedy and 100% inspirational. The book is an honest sharing of the ups and downs of **an unexpected event** in the Walker family.

Shaken to the **very roots** of their faith, Jim & Renée and their family, found healing as they successfully grappled with every **parent's worst nightmare**.

Travel along with them as they experience the roller coaster ride of tragedy, love, hope and faith, growing up with Jessica. **You will emerge touched and inspired.**

204 pages (5.5 x 8.5 inches) **ISBN 978-0-9800641-0-0**

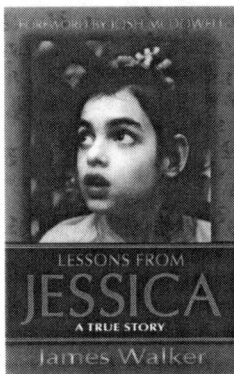

'Growing Up
with JESSICA'
Second Edition
©July 2009

'Lessons from JESSICA'

After publishing **'Growing up with Jessica.'** many readers began asking questions about the full spectrum and many **different facets** of our experience. At first we published a newsletter and then that newsletter evolved into this book.

It is designed to be a resource and guide, about the things we learned as we **'grew up with Jessica.'** At the end of each chapter are a few **'Questions for Further Thought'** and a **'Love-in-Action Point'** to help **apply the concepts**.

A **comforting**, encouraging, and enlightening book, for those facing life changing **affliction**, including their **friends and family**, who want to **be there** for them.

204 pages (5.5 x 8.5 inches) **ISBN 978-0-9800641-1-7**

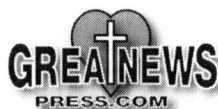

'Lessons from
JESSICA'
© 2011

GREATNEWS PRESS.COM

Our Mission:

Our mission and purpose is to offer books that do more than just motivate men, women and children... but **inspire** them. Inspiration takes many forms and has many applications.

" ...the action or power of moving the intellect or emotions..."
...the act of influencing or suggesting opinions..."

Inspirational Books by GreatNewsPress.com

CPSIA information can be obtained at www.ICGtesting.com
Printed in the USA
LVOW09s1845210214

374706LV00003B/195/P

9 780980 064186